Coloring Atlas
of the Human Body

Coloring Atlas
of the Human Body

Kerry L. Hull, BSc, PhD
Professor
Department of Biology
Bishop's University
Sherbrooke, Quebec
Canada

Wolters Kluwer | Lippincott Williams & Wilkins
Health
Philadelphia · Baltimore · New York · London
Buenos Aires · Hong Kong · Sydney · Tokyo

Acquisitions Editor: David Troy
Managing Editor: Renee Thomas
Marketing Manager: Allison Noplock
Project Manager: Rosanne Hallowell
Design Coordinator: Teresa Mallon
Production Services: Aptara, Inc.

351 West Camden Street   530 Walnut Street
Baltimore, MD 21201   Philadelphia, PA 19106

Printed in China

9 8 7 6 5 4 3 2 1

Library of Congress Cataloging-in-Publication Data

Hull, Kerry L.
   Coloring atlas of the human body / Kerry L. Hull.
       p. ; cm.
   Includes bibliographical references and index.
   ISBN 978-0-7817-6530-5 (alk. paper)
   1. Human anatomy—Atlases.   2. Human physiology—Atlases.   3. Coloring
books. I. Title.
   [DNLM: 1. Anatomy—Atlases.   2. Anatomy—Problems and Exercises.
3. Physiology—Atlases.   4. Physiology—Problems and Exercises. QS 17
H913c 2010]
QM25.H835 2010
611—dc22

                                                          2008050771

DISCLAIMER

   Care has been taken to confirm the accuracy of the information present and to describe generally ac-
cepted practices. However, the authors, editors, and publisher are not responsible for errors or omissions or
for any consequences from application of the information in this book and make no warranty, expressed or
implied, with respect to the currency, completeness, or accuracy of the contents of the publication. Application of this information in a particular situation remains the professional responsibility of the practitioner; the
clinical treatments described and recommended may not be considered absolute and universal recommendations.
   The authors, editors, and publisher have exerted every effort to ensure that drug selection and dosage
set forth in this text are in accordance with the current recommendations and practice at the time of publication. However, in view of ongoing research, changes in government regulations, and the constant flow of
information relating to drug therapy and drug reactions, the reader is urged to check the package insert for
each drug for any change in indications and dosage and for added warnings and precautions. This is particularly important when the recommended agent is a new or infrequently employed drug.
   Some drugs and medical devices presented in this publication have Food and Drug Administration
(FDA) clearance for limited use in restricted research settings. It is the responsibility of the health care
provider to ascertain the FDA status of each drug or device planned for use in their clinical practice.
   To purchase additional copies of this book, call our customer service department at **(800) 638-3030** or
fax orders to **(301) 223-2320**. International customers should call **(301) 223-2300**.
   Visit Lippincott Williams & Wilkins on the Internet: http://www.lww.com. Lippincott Williams & Wilkins
customer service representatives are available from 8:30 am to 6:00 pm, EST.

I dedicate this book to my children, Lauren and Evan.

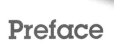
Coloring Atlas of the Human Body provides a comprehensive overview of human anatomy and physiology for visually oriented and kinesthetic learners. This atlas is not a traditional textbook; it requires active input from the reader. By coloring a series of specially designed diagrams and the accompanying flashcards, students will learn and remember concepts much more effectively than with traditional textbooks alone. The completed coloring exercises and flashcards can also serve as tools to review and prepare for examinations.

This book is particularly suited to students taking their first 3-credit course in anatomy and physiology. *Coloring Atlas of the Human Body* is a valuable supplement to any anatomy and physiology text, but can also serve as a stand-alone text.

Why Color?

Coloring is an excellent way to learn about the structure (anatomy) and function (physiology) of the human body. Anatomy, by its nature, is learned primarily by memorization. Coloring helps students remember because they must pay attention to detail, visualize structures, and physically feel the relationship between different structures as they color. Physiology builds upon anatomical knowledge by explaining how structures accomplish particular tasks. Learning physiology requires some memorization, which is facilitated by the coloring process, but it also requires an additional level of conceptual understanding. Complex pathways and principles must be broken down into component parts and subsequently reassembled and related to other pathways. Students using the *Coloring Atlas of the Human Body* approach will deepen their understanding of physiology because they can visualize the participation of structures and components in the pathway. Moreover, the necessity of coloring one section of a diagram at a time helps students to break the pathways into their component parts. Once a pathway is understood as a function of its parts and as a whole, its relevance to disease can also be understood.

Best of all, coloring is *fun* for students—a welcome distraction from more static studying activities such as reading and memorizing!

Organization

Coloring Atlas of the Human Body follows the systems approach favored by traditional anatomy and physiology textbooks, so it can be used with any such book. The first chapter summarizes fundamental concepts in anatomy, cell biology, and histology. Students will find it useful to complete these exercises before proceeding with the rest of the book. Subsequent chapters deal with the anatomy and physiology of different body systems, and need not be completed in order.

Some chapters also discuss selected aspects of disease. Sometimes, the normal functioning of a system can be best understood by studying the problems caused by disease. The effects of insulin, for example, are brought to life by learning about diabetes mellitus.

Each exercise contains two parts: a narrative page and a figure page. The narrative page summarizes critical information using bulleted lists, tables, and flowcharts, and directs the reader to the matching flashcards (if any) in Appendix I. As students read through the narrative, they will be asked to color in relevant structure names and the structures themselves on the diagram on the facing page. The action of coloring the structure name and the structure will help students remember the spelling and location of the structure. In addition, the completed diagram will serve as a useful reference and review tool, since it will be easy to match different structures to the different terms.

Flashcards

Some coloring exercises cover content students often have trouble remembering. These exercises have accompanying flashcards that can be found at the back of the book in Appendix I. The front of each flashcard features a magnified view of a section of the coloring exercise figure with up to 15 labeled structures, with the names of the structures featured on the back. Students can rip out flashcards that accompany a particular exercise and color them in conjunction with the larger figure, using the same color scheme. In addition to the extra reinforcement that coloring the flashcards provides, students benefit from being able to use the colored-in flashcards anywhere—on the bus or walking to class—as a portable study tool for review and self-testing.

Additional Student Resources

For students who have purchased the book, *Coloring Atlas of the Human Body* also includes two bonus Coloring Exercises as well as helpful study tips, available on the companion website at www.thepoint.com/HullColoringAtlas. See the inside front cover of this text for more details, including the passcode you will need to gain access to the website.

In short, the *Coloring Atlas of the Human Body* provides an essential learning package for today's visually oriented students. It integrates two popular and effective learning tools—coloring guides and flashcards—to help students learn challenging concepts and evaluate their progress.

Acknowledgments

I would like to thank Barbara Cohen, author of *Memmler's Human Body in Health and Disease* and *Memmler's Structure and Function of the Human Body*, for her tremendous leadership and support as I began my forays into textbook writing.

A number of individuals at LWW were instrumental in this project, including David Troy, John Goucher, Dana Knighten, and Renee Thomas. Enormous thanks are due to Jennifer Clements and to the artists at Dragonfly Media Group, who were able to turn my rough sketches into instructive and attractive drawings. I would also like to acknowledge the reviewers, whose feedback and suggestions were invaluable.

Finally, I thank my husband, Norman Jones, for his unstinting support and willingness to take on many household tasks, and my parents, Bill and Lorraine Hull, who always incouraged my interest in all things biomedical.

Contents

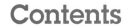

Coloring Atlas
of the Human Body

CHAPTER 1

Fundamentals of Anatomy and Physiology

Coloring Exercise 1-1 ➤ **Organ Systems and Levels of Organization**

Levels of Organization

- **Chemicals** Ⓐ
  - Basic elements (e.g., sodium, calcium) or
  - Combinations of elements
    - Carbohydrates (e.g., sugars) – Fats (e.g., cholesterol)
    - Proteins – Nucleic acids (DNA, RNA)
- **Cells** Ⓑ—see Coloring Exercise 1-4
  - Contain organelles
  - Constructed from chemicals
- **Tissues** Ⓒ—see Coloring Exercises 1-7 and 1-8
  - Specialized groups of cells
  - Epithelial, connective, nervous, and muscle tissues
- **Organs** Ⓓ—tissues functioning together
- **Systems** Ⓔ
  - Group of organs working together for the same general purpose
  - Some organs are found in several systems
- **Organism** Ⓕ systems cooperate to maintain and propagate organism

Body Systems

System	Structures	Major Functions
Integumentary	Skin and associated structures	Protection (chemical, mechanical)
Skeletal	Bones, ligaments, joints	Movement
Muscular Ⓖ	Skeletal and smooth muscles	Movement
Nervous Ⓗ	Neurons and ganglia; brain, spinal cord, and nerves	Communication
Endocrine Ⓘ	Glands	Communication
Cardiovascular Ⓙ	Heart, blood vessels	Transportation (gases, nutrients, wastes, heat)
Lymphatic Ⓚ	Lymphatic vessels, lymph nodes, tonsils, thymus, spleen	Protection (immune defense)
Respiratory Ⓛ	Lungs and respiratory tract	Gas exchange (take in oxygen, expel carbon dioxide)
Digestive	Mouth, esophagus, stomach, intestine, liver, pancreas	Extraction of usable nutrients from ingested food
Urinary Ⓜ	Kidneys, ureter, bladder, urethra	Expulsion of waste and excess water
Reproductive	External sex organs, gonads, internal duct systems	Production of offspring

✎ COLORING INSTRUCTIONS

Color each figure part and its name at the same time, using the same color. Color the six different levels of organization (parts Ⓐ to Ⓕ).

✎ COLORING INSTRUCTIONS

Color some examples of organs belonging to specific systems (parts Ⓖ to Ⓜ). Color the corresponding terms at the same time, using the same color. Note that you already colored the digestive system, and that the respiratory and urinary systems are shown on the same torso.

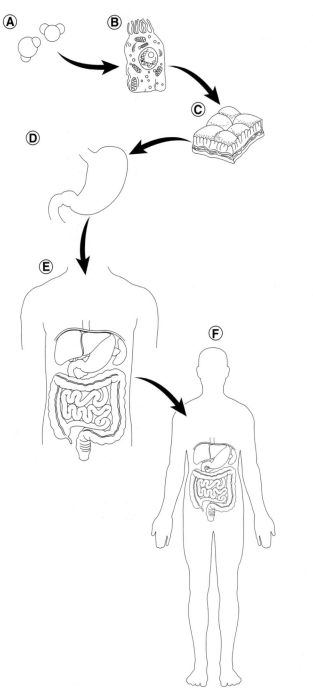
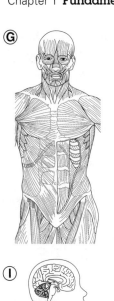
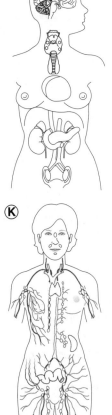
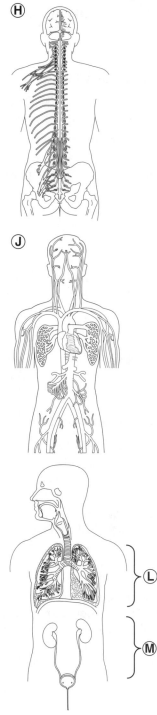

A. chemical
B. cell
C. tissue
D. organ
E. system
F. organism

G. muscular system
H. nervous system
I. endocrine system
J. cardiovascular system
K. lymphatic system
L. respiratory system
M. urinary system

Coloring Exercise 1-2 ➤ Directional Terms and Planes of Division

Directional Terms

- Terms apply to body in anatomic position (upright, face front, arms at sides, palms forward, feet parallel)
- Terms describe position of one structure in relation to another

Term	Opposite Term	Example
Ⓐ **Superior:** above	Ⓑ **Inferior:** below	Lungs are superior to intestines; intestines are inferior to lungs
Ⓐ **Cranial:** closer to head	Ⓑ **Caudal:** closer to "tail" (sacrum)	Nose is cranial to mouth; mouth is caudal to nose
Ⓒ **Ventral/Anterior:** closer to front (belly)	Ⓓ **Dorsal/Posterior:** closer to back	Sternum is ventral to vertebrae; vertebrae are dorsal to sternum
Ⓔ **Proximal:** closer to origin	Ⓕ **Distal:** farther from origin	Knee is proximal to ankle; ankle is distal to knee
Ⓖ **Medial:** closer to midline	Ⓗ **Lateral:** farther from midline	Nose is medial to ears; ears are lateral to nose

COLORING INSTRUCTIONS

On the top figure: color each arrow (representing Ⓐ to Ⓗ) and its corresponding term at the same time, using the same color.

Planes of Division

- **Frontal** plane Ⓘ
  - Longitudinal plane, in line with ears
  - Divides body into unequal anterior and posterior sections
  - Sections along this plane called longitudinal or coronal (not shown)
- **Sagittal** plane Ⓙ
  - Longitudinal plane, perpendicular to ears
  - Divides body into right and left portions
  - Sections along this plane called **longitudinal** or **sagittal** Ⓚ
  - Midsagittal section: cut body down midline
- **Transverse** plane Ⓛ
  - Divides body into unequal upper and lower segments
  - Also called horizontal plane
  - Sections along this plane called **transverse** or **cross** sections Ⓜ
  - Angled sections called **oblique** sections Ⓝ

COLORING INSTRUCTIONS

On the bottom figure: color the three planes (Ⓘ, Ⓙ, Ⓛ) and the types of sections (Ⓚ, Ⓜ, Ⓝ) the same color as the corresponding terms in the list.

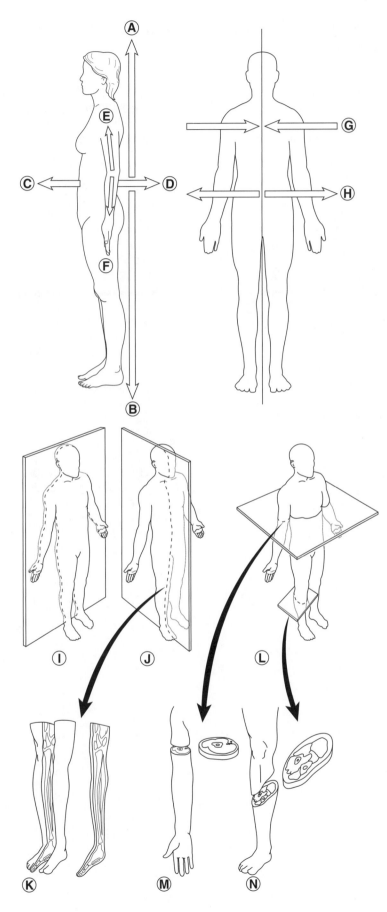

A. superior/cranial
B. inferior/caudal
C. anterior/ventral
D. posterior/dorsal
E. proximal
F. distal
G. medial
H. lateral
I. frontal/coronal
J. sagittal
K. longitudinal section
L. transverse/horizontal
M. cross-section
N. oblique section

Coloring Exercise 1-3 ➤ Body Cavities and Abdominal Regions

Body Cavities

- Body organs contained within CAVITIES (large spaces)
- Cavities lined with bone (dorsal cavities) or membranes (ventral cavities)

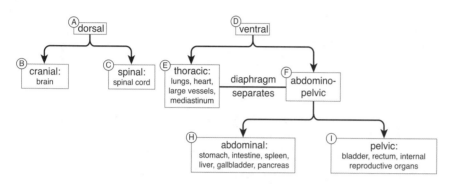

Abdominal Regions

Remember that right and left refer to the PATIENT'S right and left, not yours!

- Abdomen divided into nine regions by four lines
  - Two horizontal lines, just inferior to ribcage and just inferior to the top of hipbones
  - Two vertical lines just medial to both nipples
- Three central regions
  - Upper: **epigastric** (J)
  - Middle: **umbilical** (K)
  - Lower: **hypogastric** (L)
- Six lateral regions
  - Upper: **right** (M)/**left** (N) **hypochondriac**
  - Middle: **right** (O)/**left** (P) **lumbar**
  - Lower: **right** (Q)/**left** (R) **iliac** (inguinal)

🖍 **COLORING INSTRUCTIONS**

Color each structure and its corresponding term at the same time, using the same color. On the top figure:

1. Use the following coloring scheme: (A), blue. (B) and (C), different blues. (D), red. (E), yellow. (F), orange. (G), brown. (H) and (I), different oranges.
2. Write the correct terms on lines (A), (D), and (F) in the appropriate color.
3. Color the parts indicated by letters (B)–(C), (E), and (G)–(I).
4. You can shade the boxes in the flowchart on this page with the appropriate color as well.

🖍 **COLORING INSTRUCTIONS**

On the bottom figure: color the nine regions of the abdomen ((J) to (R)).

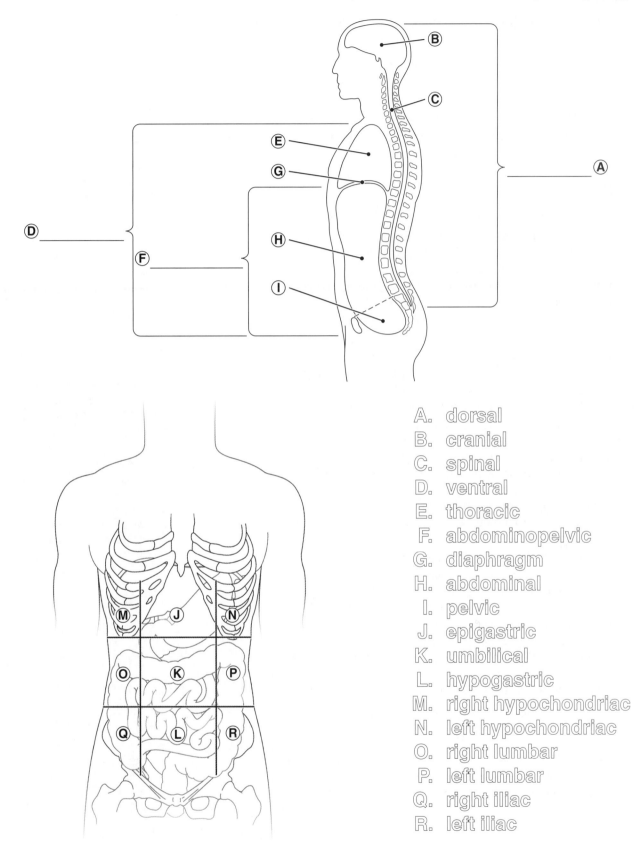

A. dorsal
B. cranial
C. spinal
D. ventral
E. thoracic
F. abdominopelvic
G. diaphragm
H. abdominal
 I. pelvic
J. epigastric
K. umbilical
L. hypogastric
M. right hypochondriac
N. left hypochondriac
O. right lumbar
P. left lumbar
Q. right iliac
R. left iliac

Coloring Exercise 1-4 ➤ Cell Structure

Cells

- Constructed from chemicals (proteins, carbohydrates, lipids, ions, water...)
- Independently carry out many life functions: energy generation, waste disposal, protein and lipid synthesis

Cell Constituents

A cell can be compared to a factory

- **Plasma membrane** (Ⓐ—see Coloring Exercise 1-5)
  - Outer wall: separates cell from its surroundings
  - Plasma membrane extensions include
    - **Cilia** Ⓑ: create fluid movement
    - **Flagellum** Ⓒ: moves entire cell (sperm cells only)

Factory Components: ORGANELLES

- Factory Library: **Nucleus** Ⓓ
  - Separated from rest of cell by the **nuclear membrane** Ⓔ
  - Contains blueprints (DNA) for all cell proteins
  - **Nucleolus** Ⓕ within nucleus assembles **ribosomes** Ⓖ
- Workers and Machines: Ribosomes/Endoplasmic reticulum
  - **Ribosomes** Ⓖ synthesize proteins from amino acids
  - **Rough endoplasmic reticulum** (ER) Ⓗ
    - Consists of ribosomes bound to membranous sacs
    - Modifies proteins synthesized by ribosomes
  - **Smooth endoplasmic reticulum** Ⓘ
    - Consists of membranous sacs without ribosomes
    - Synthesizes lipids
- Shipping and Receiving: **Golgi apparatus** Ⓙ
  - Layers of membrane-bound compartments
  - Modify, sort, and package proteins for export
  - Incoming and outgoing material packaged in **vesicles** Ⓚ
- Power Generation and Maintenance
  - **Mitochondria** Ⓛ generate energy (ATP) from nutrients
  - **Lysosomes** Ⓜ dispose of waste generated inside the cell or imported in vesicles
  - **Peroxisomes** Ⓝ break down toxic metabolic byproducts
- New Factory Development: **Centrioles** Ⓞ
  - Help organized microtubules, which move chromosomes

The Factory Air: Cytosol Ⓟ

- Contains free ribosomes, enzymes, cytoskeleton, ions, nutrients, gases, and other soluble substances

COLORING INSTRUCTIONS

Color the plasma membrane Ⓐ and the membrane extensions Ⓑ and Ⓒ different shades of yellow. Color the terms in the list the same shades.

COLORING INSTRUCTIONS

1. Color each organelle as you read about its function. Color the terms in the list in matching colors.
2. Save a light color for the cytosol Ⓟ.
3. Draw a cartoon illustrating the function of each of the organelles for Ⓓ, Ⓖ–Ⓘ, Ⓚ, Ⓛ, and Ⓜ/Ⓝ in the small boxes provided. For instance, you could draw a book for Ⓓ.

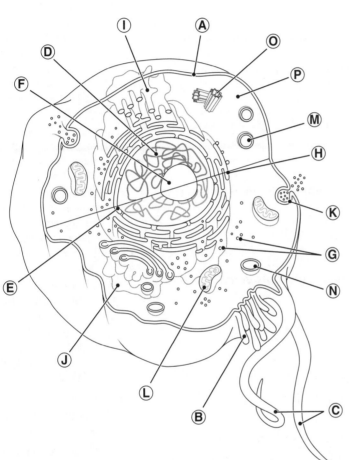
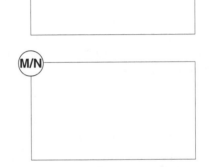

A. plasma membrane
B. cilia
C. flagellum
D. nucleus
E. nuclear membrane
F. nucleolus
G. ribosomes
H. rough endoplasmic reticulum
I. smooth endoplasmic reticulum

J. Golgi apparatus
K. vesicle
L. mitochondria
M. lysosome
N. peroxisome
O. centriole
P. cytosol

Coloring Exercise 1-5 ➤ The Plasma Membrane and Chromosomes

Plasma Membrane

Lipid bilayer separating the cytoplasm from the extracellular fluid.

Lipids (fats)

- **Phospholipid bilayer**
  - Hydrophilic **phosphate** heads Ⓐ interact with water, hydrophobic **lipid** tails Ⓑ hate water
  - Hydrophilic substances (ions, sugars, proteins) can't pass through hydrophobic membrane core
- **Cholesterol** Ⓒ
  - Lipid molecules interspersed between phospholipids that strengthen plasma membrane

Proteins

Proteins Ⓓ serve diverse functions, including **channels** Ⓔ, transporters (see Coloring Exercise 1-6), enzymes, receptors

Carbohydrates (sugars)

- Confined to the extracellular face of the membrane
- Attached to some proteins and lipids, resulting in **glycoproteins** Ⓕ and **glycolipids** Ⓖ (respectively)

Chromosomes and DNA

Chromosomes Ⓗ

- Usually unravelled; only visible during cell division
- Contain DNA and proteins. Proteins organize the DNA.

Genes Ⓘ

- Many **genes** Ⓘ in each chromosome (the figure is simplified).
- Each gene contains the information (**DNA** Ⓙ) to make a specific protein (for instance, insulin).

DNA Ⓙ

- Each gene consists of a segment of DNA Ⓙ.
- DNA consists of two strands of nucleotides.
- The sequence of nucleotides determines the sequence of the protein.

Nucleotide

- All nucleotides contain identical **phosphate** Ⓚ and **sugar** Ⓛ units: these make up the DNA backbone
- Each nucleotide contains one of four nitrogen bases: **guanine** (G) Ⓜ, **cytosine** (C) Ⓝ, **adenine** (A) Ⓞ, **thymine** (T) Ⓟ
- Nitrogen bases give nucleotides their identity and bind the two DNA strands together
- A binds T, G binds C

COLORING INSTRUCTIONS

Color each structure and its name at the same time, using the same color. On the top figure:

1. Color phospholipid heads Ⓐ dark blue and tails Ⓑ light blue in the magnified phospholipid and in the membrane.

2. Find and color the cholesterol molecules Ⓒ red. They have smaller heads and shorter, uneven tails.

3. Try to find and color all examples of each part. For instance, color all of the phospholipid heads, not just the labelled ones.

4. Color the channel dark purple and the other proteins light purple.

5. Color the sugar molecules attached to proteins Ⓕ and lipids Ⓖ, using light and dark pink.

COLORING INSTRUCTIONS

On the bottom figure:

1. Shade the entire chromosome Ⓗ light yellow.

2. Color the different boxes on the chromosome, representing different genes, a rainbow of colors. Color the boxed gene Ⓘ light green.

3. Color the DNA Ⓙ in the box brown.

4. Color the phosphate Ⓚ and sugar Ⓛ units light and dark brown (respectively)

5. Color the guanine Ⓜ and thymine Ⓟ bases, and the labelled cytosine Ⓝ and thymine Ⓟ bases.

6. Can you determine the identity of the other bases? Color them.

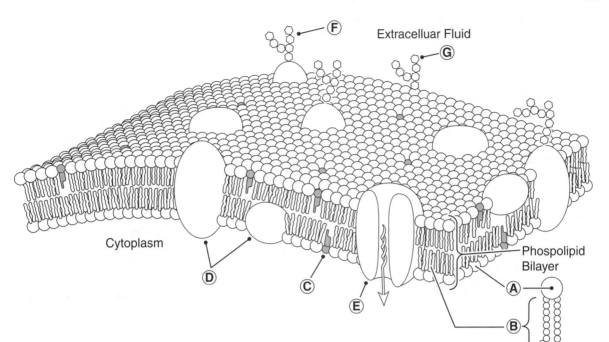

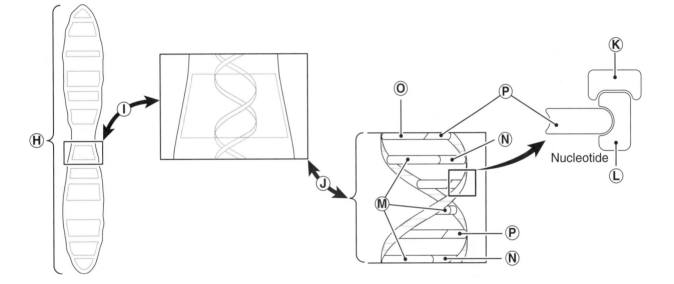

A. phospholipid head (phosphate)
B. phospholipid tail (lipid)
C. cholesterol
D. membrane protein
E. protein channel
F. glycoprotein
G. glycolipid

H. chromosome
I. gene
J. DNA segment
K. phosphate unit
L. sugar unit
M. guanine
N. cytosine
O. adenine
P. thymine

Coloring Exercise 1-6 ➤ Membrane Transport

Concentration Gradients and Transport

- The top figure shows the distribution of a **solute** (circles, Ⓐ) dissolved in **water** (squares, Ⓑ) in the cytosol and extracellular fluid. The solute can pass between the **membrane phospholipids** Ⓒ.
- More solute = less water
- Solute concentration gradient (large left arrow) directed into cell (there are more circles outside than inside)
- **Diffusion** Ⓓ: NET influx of circles, with the gradient
  - Kinetic energy of solute particles drives movement; no ATP required
  - Circles will enter and exit cell, but more will enter cell
- **Active transport** Ⓔ: efflux of circles with the help of **ATP** Ⓕ, against the gradient.
- **Osmosis** Ⓖ: NET movement of water out of cell, with the water (osmotic) gradient. Water cannot be actively transported.
- Substances also enter and exit cells by other mechanisms (exocytosis, endocytosis, pinocytosis, phagocytosis; not shown).

Transport Mechanisms

Determined by the DIRECTION of the concentration gradient and the PERMEABILITY of the membrane

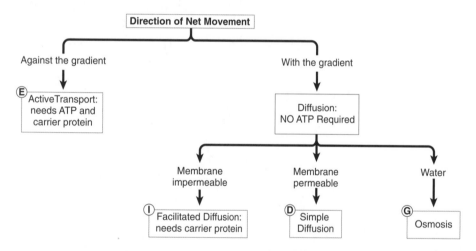

Carrier Proteins

Carrier proteins Ⓗ

- Required for **facilitated diffusion** Ⓘ and **active transport** Ⓔ
- Conformational changes in protein move substance through plasma membrane
  - Import particle: begin with conformation 1 and end with conformation 3
  - Export particle: begin with conformation 3 and end with conformation 1
- Facilitated diffusion: transporters work in both directions, but net movement is with gradient
- Active transport: transporter works in one direction (against gradient); ATP required for conformational change

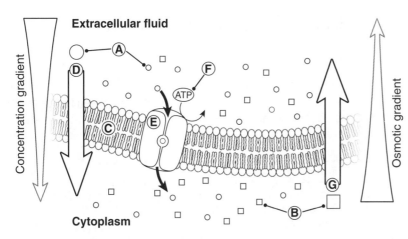

A.   solute
B.   water
C.   membrane
      phospholipids
D.   diffusion
E.   active transport
F.   ATP
G.   osmosis
H.   carrier protein
 I.   facilitated
      diffusion

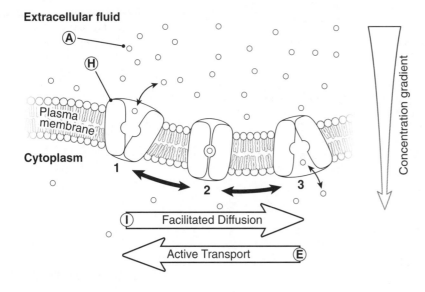

Coloring Exercise 1-7 ➤ Tissues 1: Epithelial Tissues

Four Tissue Types

- Tissues contain living **cells** (Ⓐ1 to Ⓓ1) and sometimes nonliving **matrix** (Ⓔ).
- Matrix can contain water, minerals, protein fibers

Tissue Type	Structure	Function
Epithelial (Ⓐ, this Coloring Exercise)	Tightly packed epithelial cells Ⓐ1 Minimal matrix No blood supply Usually attached to adjacent connective tissue by **basement membrane** Ⓕ	*Protective*: Lines inner cavities and blood vessels, covers outer surface *Secretory*: Forms endocrine/exocrine glands *Transport*: regulates movement between cells and body cavities/blood
Muscle (Ⓑ, Coloring Exercise 4-1)	Tightly packed **muscle cells** Ⓑ1 Minimal matrix	Movement
Nervous (Ⓒ, Coloring Exercise 5-2)	**Neurons** Ⓒ1, glia	Conduct nerve impulses
Connective (Ⓓ, Coloring Exercise 1-7)	Cells (e.g., **fibroblast** Ⓓ1) separated by large amounts of **matrix** Ⓔ Matrix ranges from liquid (blood) to hard (bone)	Supports all parts of the body Specialized functions (blood, bone)

Classification of Epithelial Tissues

Classified by number of layers, cell appearance

Number of Layers

- **Simple** Ⓖ to Ⓘ: one layer resting on basement membrane, easy passage of chemicals and gases
- **Stratified** Ⓙ: multiple layers, stronger
- **Pseudostratified** Ⓚ: stratified appearance, but single layer of staggered cells

Cell Appearance

- **Squamous** Ⓖ: flat, irregular
- **Cuboidal** Ⓗ: square
- **Columnar** Ⓘ: long and narrow
- **Transitional:** cells can compress and expand (not shown)

✎ **COLORING INSTRUCTIONS**
Color each structure and its name at the same time, using the same color. On the top figure:

1. Color the cells (Ⓐ1 to Ⓓ1) in the different tissue types different colors. Note the wide variety of cell shapes.
2. Color the **basement membrane** (Ⓕ) for the epithelial tissue.
3. Color the **matrix** (Ⓔ) for the connective tissue. Other tissues have minimal matrix.

✎ **COLORING INSTRUCTIONS**
On the bottom figure:

1. Color the basement membrane gray in each picture. It has been labelled for you in picture Ⓖ.
2. Color the cells in each type of epithelia (Ⓖ to Ⓚ) in different colors.

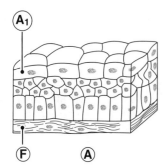

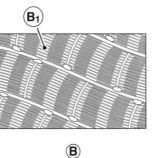

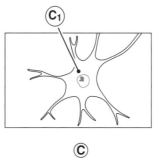

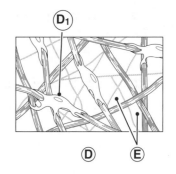

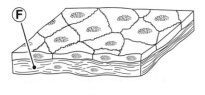

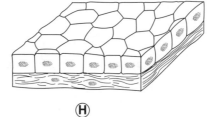

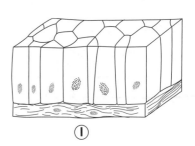

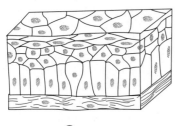

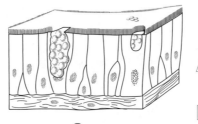

A. epithelial tissue
A₁. epithelial cells
B. muscle tissue
B₁. muscle cells
C. nervous tissue
C₁. neuron
D. connective tissue
D₁. fibroblast
E. matrix
F. basement membrane
G. squamous
H. cuboidal
I. columar
J. stratified
K. pseudostratified

Coloring Exercise 1-8 ➤ Tissues 2: Connective Tissues

Characteristics of Connective Tissue

- Constitutes the connective fabric of the body
- Cells separated by nonliving matrix
- Matrix can be liquid, jellylike, fibrous, or hard
- Matrix components can include water, protein fibers, minerals

Classification of Connective Tissue

Determined by distribution and function

Type	Example	Cells	Matrix	Functions
Circulating: fluid consistency	**Blood** Ⓐ	**Blood cells** Ⓐ1	**Plasma** Ⓑ	Transport of nutrients, gases, waste
	Lymph (not shown)	Leukocytes	Lymph	Immune defense, fat transport
Generalized: widely distributed	**Adipose** Ⓒ	**Adipose cells** Ⓒ1	Minimal: Cells contain **fat droplets** Ⓓ	Cushions joints Heat insulator Energy supply
	Areolar Ⓔ	**Fibroblasts** Ⓔ1 **Immune cells** Ⓕ	**Collagen** Ⓖ & **elastic fibers** Ⓗ: Jellylike **background substance** Ⓘ Contains c**apillaries** Ⓙ	Most abundant tissue Surrounds vessels/organs Supports, nourishes skin Separates muscle sheaths
	Tendons Ⓚ, ligaments (not shown)	**Fibroblasts** Ⓚ1	Densely packed **collagen** Ⓖ, elastic fibers (not shown): Fibrous matrix	Connect muscles (tendons) or bones (ligaments) to bones
Structural: associated with the skeleton	**Cartilage** Ⓛ	**Chondrocytes** Ⓛ1	Firm **matrix** Ⓜ	Shock absorption Reduces friction in joints Provides shape (e.g., nose)
	Bone Ⓝ	**Osteocytes** Ⓝ1, osteoblasts	Mineral **matrix** Ⓞ	See Coloring Exercise 3-1

✎ COLORING INSTRUCTIONS

Color each structure and its name at the same time, using the same color. Read all instructions before proceeding.

1. Choose six contrasting colors for the six connective tissues shown in the figure.
2. Use these colors to lightly shade the relevant table rows.
3. Use the same colors for the cells of each tissue. For example, color blood cells Ⓐ1 the color used for blood Ⓐ.
4. Color the matrix of each tissue, using a color related to the one used for the cells. For instance, use dark red for Ⓐ1 and light pink for Ⓑ.
5. Note that some components (e.g., collagen) are found in more than one tissue type.

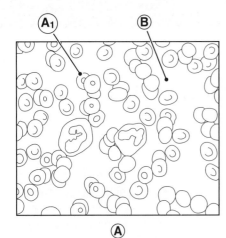

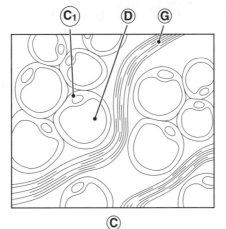

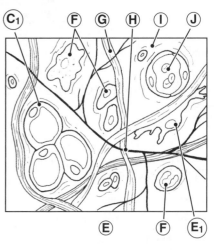

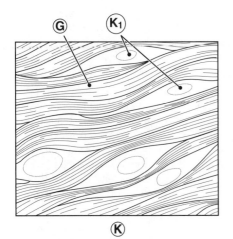

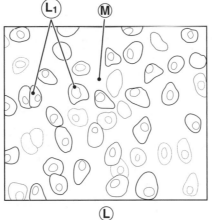

A.   blood
A₁. blood cells
B.   plasma
C.   adipose tissue
C₁. adipose cell
D.   fat droplet
E.   areolar tissue

E₁. fibroblast (areolar)
F.   mast cell
G.   collagen
H.   elastic fiber
I.   jelly-like substance
J.   capillary
K.   tendon

K₁. fibroblast (tendon)
L.   cartilage
L₁. chondrocyte
M.   cartilage matrix
N.   bone
N₁. osteocyte
O.   mineral matrix

CHAPTER 2

The Skin

Coloring Exercise 2-1 ➤ Skin Structure and Function

Skin Functions

- Protection against infection, dehydration, cold, heat
- Sensory information collection
- Vitamin D synthesis

Skin Structure

Skin Layer	Structure	Characteristics	Function
Epidermis Ⓐ		Surface portion of skin; no blood vessels	Separates body from the environment
	Stratum corneum Ⓓ	Surface layer; keratin-filled cells	Protective layer
	Stratum basale Ⓔ	Deepest epidermal layer	Produces new epidermal cells
	Melanocyte	Cell deep within epidermis	Produces melanin
Dermis Ⓑ		Connective tissue; many **blood vessels** Ⓕ and **nerves** Ⓖ	Cushions, stretches
Subcutaneous Layer Ⓒ		Connective tissue under skin; contains **adipose tissue** Ⓗ	Connects skin to surface muscle; insulates; stores energy
Accessory Structures	**Pressure receptor** Ⓘ	Distends in response to pressure, activating sensory nerve	Detects pressure
	Touch receptor Ⓙ	Distends in response to touch, activating nerve	Detects light touch
	Free nerve endings Ⓖ1		Detect pain, temperature
	Sebaceous (oil) **glands** Ⓚ	Associated with hair follicles; produce sebum	Sebum lubricates skin; prevents dehydration
	Eccrine sudoriferous glands Ⓛ	Gland secretes watery, salty sweat via a **pore** Ⓛ1	Cooling
	Hair Ⓜ	Grows from **hair follicle** Ⓜ1; **arrector pili** muscle Ⓝ elevates hair	Heat conservation, protection from ultraviolet light
	Nails	Composed of keratin synthesized by stratum corneum cells	Protect fingers and toes; facilitate grasping

✎ COLORING INSTRUCTIONS

Color each structure and its name at the same time, using the same color.

1. Color the names of the skin layers (Ⓐ to Ⓒ). Use red for epidermis, blue for dermis, and yellow for subcutaneous layer.

2. As you read through the table, color each structure as you review its characteristics and function. Try to color all examples of each structure (for instance, all of the nerves).

3. Use variants of red for the epidermal layers.

4. Shade the background connective tissue in the dermis light blue.

5. Color the adipose tissue Ⓗ light yellow.

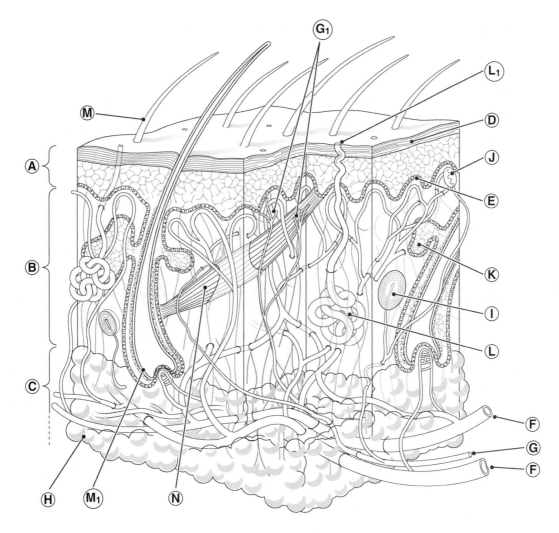

A. epidermis
B. dermis
C. subcutaneous layer
D. stratum corneum
E. stratum basale
F. blood vessels
G. nerves
G_1. free nerve endings
H. adipose tissue

I. pressure receptor
J. touch receptor
K. sebaceous gland
L. eccrine sudoriferous gland
L_1. pore
M. hair
M_1. hair follicle
N. arrector pili muscle

Coloring Exercise 2-2 ➤ Skin Disorders

Common Skin Lesions

- Classified by size, firmness, appearance, and the presence/absence of fluid
- Caused by disease, drugs, physical trauma
- Rash: temporary skin eruption

Lesion	Definition	Examples
SURFACE LESIONS		
Macule Ⓓ	Small spot neither raised nor depressed. Larger area called *patch*	Freckles, measles
Papule Ⓔ	Small firm, raised area. Larger areas called *nodules*	Some chicken pox, pimple, mole
Vesicle Ⓕ	Small blister filled with serous fluid. Larger blisters called *bullae*	Shingles, herpes simplex
Pustule Ⓖ	Pus-filled vesicle	Infected vesicle, acne, impetigo
DEEP LESIONS		
Excoriation	Scratch	
Laceration	Rough, jagged wound	
Ulcer Ⓗ	Open sore caused by tissue disintegration	Bedsore
Fissure Ⓘ	Skin crack	Athlete's foot

Burns

- Caused by chemicals, abrasion, sunlight, contact with hot objects or liquids
- Classified by depth of damage, surface area involved

Depth of Tissue Damage

Classification	Skin Layers Involved	Appearance	Examples
Superficial partial-thickness	Epidermis, occasionally part of dermis	Reddened skin; possibly blisters	Sunburn
Deep partial-thickness	Epidermis, part of dermis	Blistered, broken skin; weeping surface	Scalding
Full-thickness	Full skin, occasionally underlying structures	Tissue may be broken, dry, and pale or charred	Requires skin grafting

Surface Area

- Estimated by Lund and Browder method (more accurate, not shown) or Rule of Nines
- Each area assigned percentage in multiples of nine (Ⓙ to Ⓝ)
- Example: burn to both **legs** Ⓝ, **external genitalia** Ⓜ covers 19% of body surface

✎ **COLORING INSTRUCTIONS**

Color each figure part and its corresponding term at the same time, using the same color. On the top figure:

1. Lightly color the three skin layers (Ⓐ to Ⓒ) in each diagram. They have been labeled for you in figure G.
2. As you go through the table, color each lesion on the diagram and photograph (Ⓓ to Ⓘ).
3. Note the skin layers implicated in each lesion.
4. You can also lightly shade each table row with the same color.

✎ **COLORING INSTRUCTIONS**

On the bottom figure: Color each body area and the relevant percentage in the anterior and posterior torsos (Ⓙ to Ⓝ).

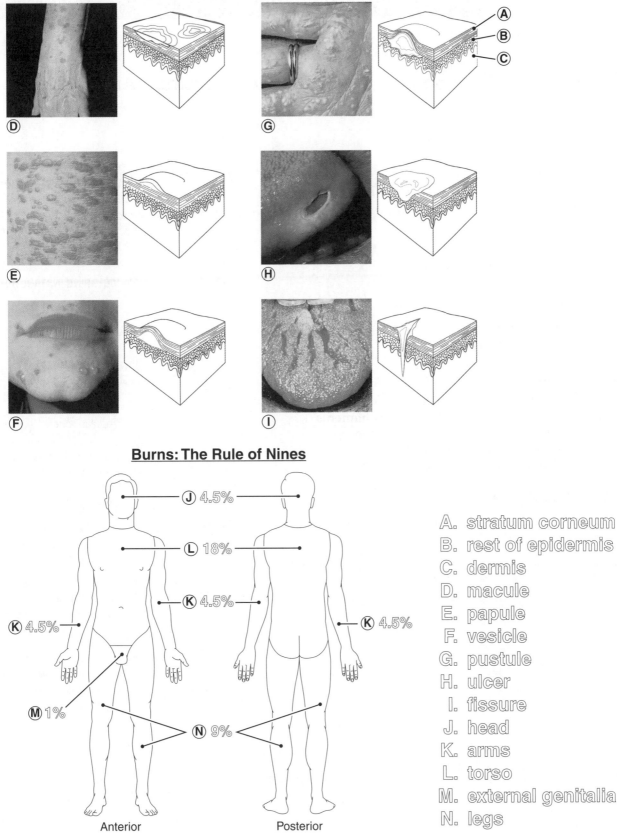

Burns: The Rule of Nines

Anterior   Posterior

A. stratum corneum
B. rest of epidermis
C. dermis
D. macule
E. papule
F. vesicle
G. pustule
H. ulcer
I. fissure
J. head
K. arms
L. torso
M. external genitalia
N. legs

CHAPTER 3

The Skeletal System

Coloring Exercise 3-1 ➤ The Skeletal System: An Overview

Skeletal Divisions

- Axial skeleton: head and trunk; 80 bones (Ⓐ to Ⓗ)
- Appendicular skeleton: 126 bones of the shoulders, hips, arms, legs (Ⓘ to Ⓩ)

Bone Functions

- Serve as body framework (all bones)
- Protect delicate structures (e.g., brain, Ⓐ)
- Work with muscles to produce movement (e.g., Ⓢ)
- Store calcium salts (all bones)
- Produce blood cells (red bone marrow)

Bone Shapes

- Bones have different shapes to accomplish different functions
  - Long bones (levers, blood cell synthesis); **humerus** Ⓚ
  - Short (joints); wrist (**carpals** Ⓝ), ankle, kneecap
  - Flat (protection); skull, ribs, **sternum** Ⓓ
  - Irregular (varied functions); **vertebrae** Ⓖ, hip bones

Bone Markings

Projections form joints (head, condyle, some processes) or sites of attachment for connective tissue (all others)

Marking	Description	Example
Process	Any raised area of bone	
Head	Rounded, knoblike end	
Condyle	Rounded projection	
Epicondyle	Small projection above condyle	
Tuberosity	Large, rounded projection	
Trochanter	Very large projection	

Depressions and holes form joints or permit the passage of soft tissue

Marking	Description	Example
Foramen (plural: foramina)	Hole permitting passage of nerve or vessel	
Sinus	Air space	
Fossa	Shallow depression on a bone surface	
Meatus	Short channel	

COLORING INSTRUCTIONS

Lightly color the bones of the axial skeleton light blue (Ⓐ–Ⓗ) and the appendicular skeleton (Ⓘ–Ⓩ) yellow.

COLORING INSTRUCTIONS

1. Color a few examples of each bone type on the skeleton in different colors.
2. Use brown for long bones, dark green for short bones, red for flat bones, and purple for irregular bones.
3. Once you have finished your study of skeletal anatomy, use this Coloring Exercise for review. Write the name of each bone in the blanks beside the skeleton. The answers are listed in Appendix I.

INSTRUCTIONS

Look through Coloring Exercises 3-6 to 3-12 to find examples of each bone marking. Write the example in the box on the table to the left. To get you started, you can find an example of an epicondyle in Coloring Exercise 3-11.

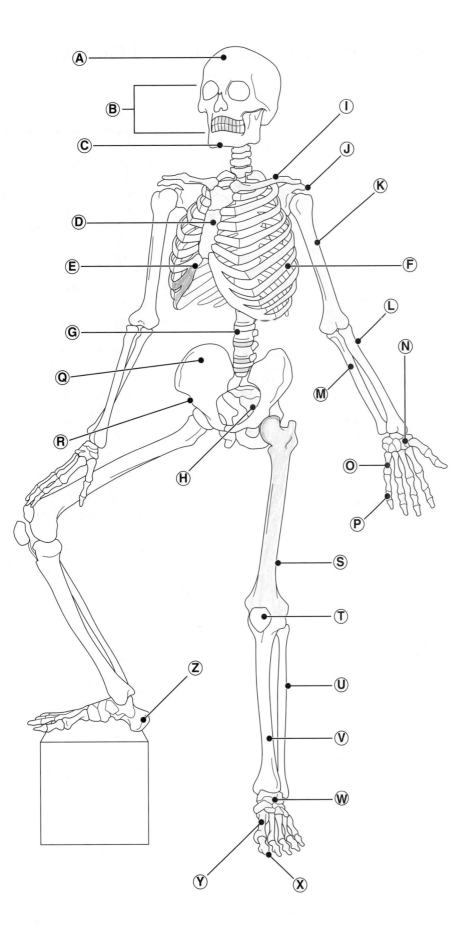
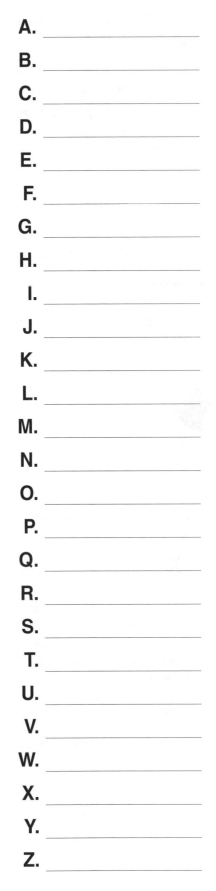

A. _____

B. _____

C. _____

D. _____

E. _____

F. _____

G. _____

H. _____

I. _____

J. _____

K. _____

L. _____

M. _____

N. _____

O. _____

P. _____

Q. _____

R. _____

S. _____

T. _____

U. _____

V. _____

W. _____

X. _____

Y. _____

Z. _____

Coloring Exercise 3-2 ➤ Long Bone Structure and Fractures

Structure of a Long Bone

- Middle shaft (**diaphysis** Ⓐ) and two irregular ends (**proximal epiphysis** Ⓑ, **distal epiphysis** Ⓒ)
- Covered by a connective tissue membrane, the **periosteum** Ⓓ
  - Periosteum contains blood vessels, nerve fibers, bone-building osteoblasts

Epiphyses Ⓑ, Ⓒ
- Contain **spongy bone** Ⓔ
  - Small, bony plates filled with red marrow
  - red marrow synthesizes blood cells
- Bones grow at the epiphyseal plate
  - When growth is complete, epiphyseal plate fuses to form the **epiphyseal line** Ⓕ

Diaphysis Ⓑ
- **Compact bone** (Ⓖ, see next exercise) surrounding a hollow space (**medullary cavity,** Ⓗ)
- **Medullary cavity**
  - Lined by **endosteum** (Ⓘ, connective tissue membrane)
  - Contains **yellow marrow** (Ⓙ, contains fat) and **blood vessels** Ⓚ

Fractures

- The most common bone lesion
- Fractures can be described by more than one term (e.g., a closed, impacted, spiral fracture)

Classification of Fractures

- Condition of skin
  - **Closed** Ⓛ: skin remains unbroken, or
  - **Open** Ⓜ: bone fragments protrude through skin
- Degree of break
  - Complete: bone completely broken, or
  - Partial: incomplete break, e.g., **greenstick** Ⓝ
- Nature of the fracture pieces
  - **Impacted** Ⓞ: bone fragments wedged together
  - **Comminuted** Ⓟ: multiple bone fragments
- Pattern of the fracture line
  - **Spiral** Ⓠ: bone twisted apart
  - **Transverse** Ⓡ: fracture line is straight across the bone
  - **Oblique** Ⓢ: fracture line is at an angle

COLORING INSTRUCTIONS

Color each structure and its name at the same time, using the same color. On the top figure:

1. Color the boxes (Ⓐ–Ⓒ) and the corresponding terms in the list with different colors. Do not use red, yellow, or brown.
2. Color the periosteum Ⓓ brown where it covers the bone.
3. Color the other parts of the long bone. Use red for Ⓔ and yellow for Ⓖ. Use very dark colors to outline Ⓕ and Ⓘ.

COLORING INSTRUCTIONS

On the bottom figure: color the bone corresponding to each fracture classification (Ⓛ to Ⓢ) and the corresponding term, using the same color.

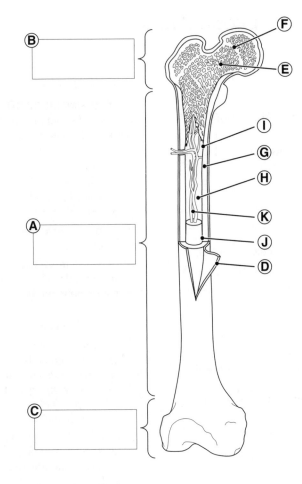

B. [   ]

A. [   ]

C. [   ]

A. diaphysis
B. proximal epiphysis
C. distal epiphysis
D. periosteum
E. spongy bone
F. epiphysial line
G. compact bone
H. medullary cavity
I. endosteum
J. yellow marrow
K. blood vessels
L. closed
M. open
N. greenstick
O. impacted
P. comminuted
Q. spiral
R. transverse
S. oblique

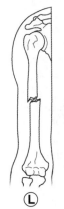

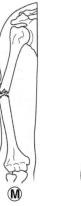

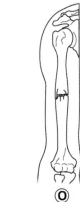

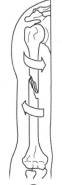

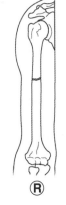

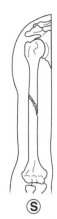

Ⓛ   Ⓜ   Ⓝ   Ⓞ   Ⓟ   Ⓠ   Ⓡ   Ⓢ

Coloring Exercise 3-3 ➤ Compact Bone Tissue

Long Bones

- Remember that long bones consist of **proximal** Ⓐ and **distal** Ⓑ **epiphyses** and a middle **diaphysis** Ⓒ
- The diaphysis consists of compact bone surrounding a **medullary cavity** Ⓓ
- Long bones are covered by the **periosteum** Ⓔ

Compact Bone Tissue

- Compact bone is HARD
  - Consists of concentric rings of **bone matrix** Ⓕ, primarily calcium salts, organized in **osteons** Ⓖ
  - Ringlike structure adds strength
- Compact bone is ALIVE
  - The diagram at the far right shows live bone
  - **Osteocytes** Ⓗ (spiderlike, living cells) maintain bone
  - Osteocytes live in spaces (**lacunae** Ⓘ) between rings of hard bone tissue
  - Osteocytes touch each other through small radiating channels (**canaliculi** Ⓙ)
  - Blood vessels nourish bone
  - **Central canal** Ⓚ, **perforating canals** Ⓛ contain **blood vessels** Ⓜ and nerves (not shown)
- The middle diagram shows dead bone; only lacunae are observed
- Remember that the central canal and medullary cavity are completely different!

✍ **COLORING INSTRUCTIONS**
Color each structure and its name at the same time, using the same color.

1. Color the epiphyses and diaphysis (Ⓐ to Ⓒ) where only the bone exterior is visible.
2. Color part Ⓓ in the small cutout.
3. Color the term "osteon" Ⓖ black; do not color the osteons on the diagrams.
4. Color the periosteum Ⓔ.
5. Color the perforating canals Ⓛ and both occurrences of the central canal Ⓚ using light colors (you can color over the vessels).
6. Color the blood vessels Ⓜ purple (each canal contains both arteries and veins).
7. Color the bone matrix Ⓕ light yellow. You may want to lightly shade the entire bone of each diagram, except the large canals, blood vessels, and periosteum.
8. Color the osteocytes Ⓗ using a dark color.
9. Color some of the lacunae Ⓘ and the canaliculi Ⓙ.

A. proximal epiphysis
B. distal epiphysis
C. diaphysis
D. medullary cavity
E. periosteum
F. bone matrix
G. osteon

H. osteocyte
I. lacunae
J. canaliculi
K. central canal
L. perforating canal
M. blood vessels

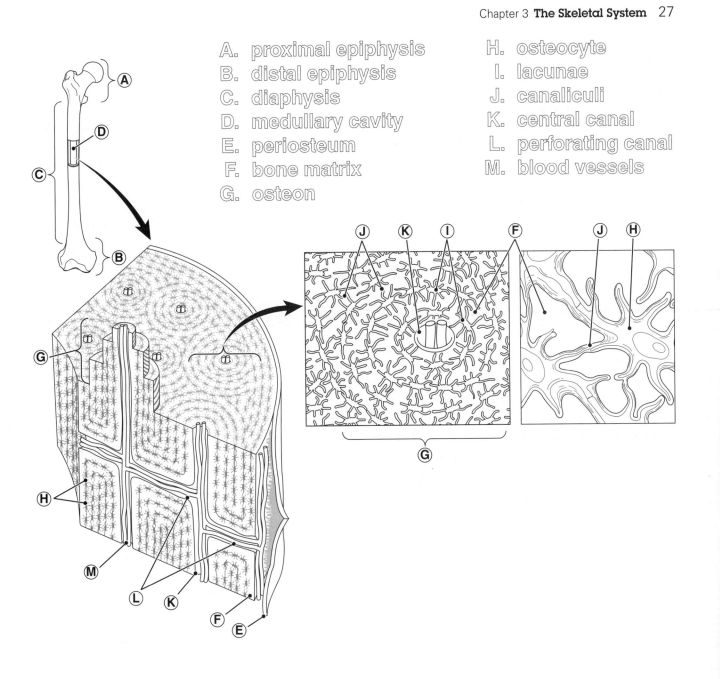

Coloring Exercise 3-4 ➤ Joints: Classification

Classification of Joints

Functional Classification: Degree of Movement

- Synarthrosis: no movement
- Amphiarthrosis: minimal movement
- Synovial: significant movement
- Higher mobility often equates with frequent injury

Structural Classification: Anatomical Characteristics

Joint Type	Characteristics	Examples
Fibrous: Usually synarthroses	No synovial cavity; bones joined by connective tissue	Skull sutures Ⓐ, syndesmosis joining radius and ulna Ⓑ
Cartilaginous: Usually amphiarthroses	No synovial cavity; bones held together by cartilage	Pubic symphysis Ⓒ; joints between vertebral bodies
Synovial: Usually diarthroses	Joint cavity: see Coloring Exercise 3-5	See below: Ⓓ to Ⓘ

Classification of Synovial Joints

Synovial joints classified by anatomy and function

Joint Type	Anatomical Characteristics	Movements Permitted	Examples
Gliding (or planar) Ⓓ	Flat or slightly curved surfaces	Gliding movements along a plane	Joints between wrist bones (Coloring Exercise 3-12)
Hinge Ⓔ	Convex surface of one bone fits into concave surface of another	Movements change the angle between bones along 1 axis	Knee joint (Coloring Exercise 3-5)
Pivot Ⓕ	Rounded surface of one bone fits into a ring created by another bone and ligament	Rotation around the length of the bone	Joint between first two neck vertebrae (rotates head); radioulnar joint (elbow; rotates forearm; Coloring Exercise 3-9)
Condyloid Ⓖ	Oval-shaped projection on bone fits into oval-shaped depression in other bone	Side-to-side and back-and-forth	Joint between finger and hand (knuckle) (Coloring Exercise 3-12); joint between skull and vertebrae
Saddle Ⓗ	Each bone has convex and concave areas	Side-to-side and back-and-forth	Joint between the thumb and the hand (Coloring Exercise 3-12)
Ball-and-socket Ⓘ	Ball-like head of one bone fits into socketlike depression of other bone	Movements in many directions	Shoulder and hip joints (Coloring Exercise 3-10)

COLORING INSTRUCTIONS

Color each illustration and its corresponding term at the same time, using the same color.

1. Color the examples of fibrous and cartilaginous joints (Ⓐ to Ⓒ). Use related colors for the two fibrous joints (Ⓐ and Ⓑ).

2. The bones are not shown for the synovial joints. Color the body part and model for each synovial joint type (Ⓓ to Ⓘ). View the anatomical characteristics of each joint type on the cross-referenced Coloring Exercises.

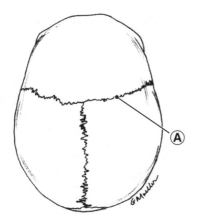

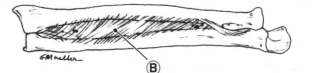

A. fibrous (suture)
B. fibrous (syndesmosis)
C. cartilagenous (symphysis)
D. synovial (gliding)
E. synovial (hinge)
F. synovial (pivot)
G. synovial (condyloid)
H. synovial (saddle)
I. synovial (ball and socket)

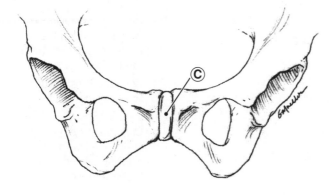

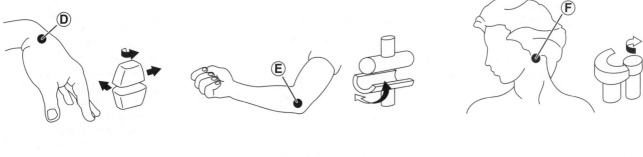

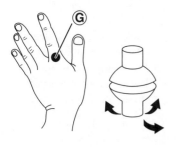

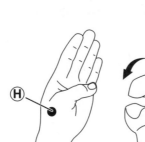

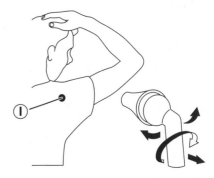

Coloring Exercise 3-5 ➤ Synovial Joints: Structure and Disease

General Characteristics

All Synovial Joints Contain

- **Joint capsule**: fibrous connective tissue continuous with periosteum encloses each joint
  - Knee joint: capsule is weak and incomplete (not shown on top figure)
  - **Synovial membrane** Ⓐ lines the capsule (but does not cover the **articular cartilage** Ⓑ)
- **Joint cavity** Ⓒ contains synovial fluid
- **Articular cartilage** Ⓑ: protects bone surfaces
- **Ligaments** Ⓓ hold bones (**femur** Ⓔ, **tibia** Ⓕ, **patella** Ⓖ) together

Some Synovial Joints Contain

- **Fat pads** Ⓗ: help protect joint
- **Bursae** (Ⓘ Ⓙ Ⓚ): small sacs containing synovial fluid; sometimes extend from the joint cavity
- Additional cartilage: cushions joint (e.g., **meniscus** Ⓛ)
- Tendons also strengthen joint (e.g., **quadriceps tendon** Ⓜ)

Arthritis

Arthritis: joint inflammation

Rheumatoid Arthritis (Bottom Center Figure)

- Usually strikes smaller joints first (like hands)
- Autoimmune disorder; antibodies attack joint tissues
- Inflammatory enzymes destroy joint cartilage and bone
- Abnormal tissue (**pannus** Ⓝ) grows in synovial membrane
  - Pannus contains inflammatory cells, many blood vessels
- Result: joint inflammation and pain, swelling, lack of mobility

Osteoarthritis (Bottom Right Figure)

- Also known as degenerative joint disease (DJD)
- Occurs mostly in weight bearing joints (e.g., knees, hips) due to normal wear and tear
- Erosion of articular cartilage, eventually bone
- New bone forms at joint margins, narrowing joint and eventually forming **bone spurs** Ⓞ
- Cartilage atrophies, ligaments calcify
- Result: limited movement

✎ COLORING INSTRUCTIONS

Color each bone and its name at the same time, using the same color. On the top figure:

1. Color the bones of the knee joint (Ⓔ to Ⓖ) using related light colors.

2. Use a dark color to outline structure Ⓐ. This thin membrane overlies structure Ⓑ.

3. Color the articular cartilage Ⓑ covering the three bones (it is labeled for the femur Ⓔ).

4. Color the joint cavity (Ⓒ, lightly shaded). A bursa Ⓘ is continuous with Ⓒ.

5. Color the other joint structures (Ⓒ, Ⓓ, Ⓗ to Ⓜ). Use related colors for the three bursae (Ⓘ Ⓙ Ⓚ).

✎ COLORING INSTRUCTIONS

Bottom three figures:

1. Color the synovial membrane Ⓐ, articular cartilage Ⓑ and joint cavity Ⓒ on the normal joint (bottom left) and the two diseased joints (bottom center and right). Note that very little normal synovial membrane remains in the joint with rheumatoid arthritis because a large pannus has formed.

2. Color the pannus Ⓝ and the bone spur Ⓞ.

3. Compare the changes in the different joint structures resulting from rheumatoid arthritis (bottom center) and osteoarthritis (bottom right).

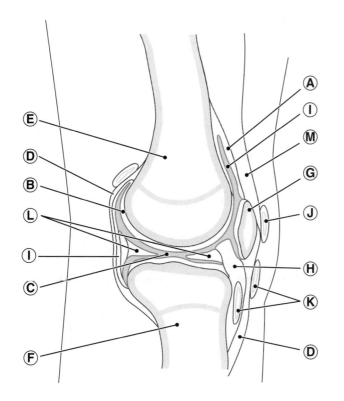

A. synovial membrane
B. articular cartilage
C. joint cavity
D. ligament
E. femur
F. tibia
G. patella
H. fat pad
 I. suprapatellar bursa
J. prepatellar bursa
K. infrapatellar bursa
L. meniscus (cartilage)
M. quadriceps tendon
N. pannus
O. bone spur

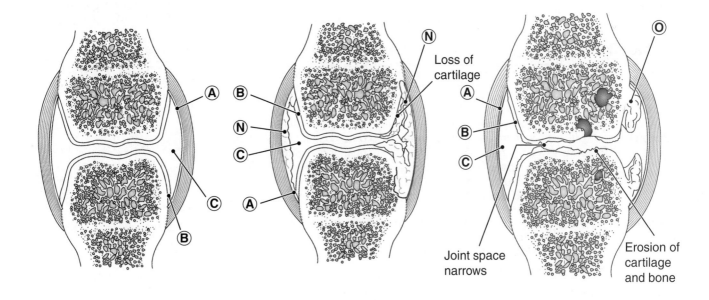

Loss of
cartilage

Joint space
narrows

Erosion of
cartilage
and bone

Coloring Exercise 3-6 ➤ The Skull

Facial Bones

Bone	Bone Features	Bone Functions
1 **Mandible** Ⓐ	Only moveable skull bone	Forms lower jaw: joint with maxilla
2 **Maxillae** (fused) Ⓑ	Contain maxillary sinus; cleft palate results if bones do not fuse	Forms upper jaw bone, part of eye orbit, nasal cavity, hard palate
2 **Zygomatic** bones Ⓒ	Articulate with temporal, maxilla, frontal, sphenoid	Form cheekbones, part of eye orbit
2 **Nasal** bones Ⓓ	Articulate with nasal cartilage	Form bridge of nose
2 **Lacrimal** bones Ⓔ	Smallest facial bones	Form part of eye orbit wall
Vomer Ⓕ	Articulates with ethmoid, palatine, maxillae	Forms inferior part of nasal septum
2 **Palatine** bones Ⓖ	L-shaped bones (not shown)	Forms part of hard palate, nasal cavity, eye orbit
2 **Inferior nasal conchae** Ⓗ	Protrude into nasal cavity	Form part of nasal cavity

Cranial Bones

Bone	Bone Features	Bone Functions
Frontal bone Ⓘ	Contains frontal sinuses	Forms forehead, eye orbit roofs, part of cranial floor
2 **Parietal** bones Ⓙ	Articulate with frontal bone (**coronal suture** Ⓚ), temporal bones (**squamous suture** Ⓛ), occipital bone (**lambdoid suture** Ⓜ), and each other (**sagittal suture** Ⓝ)	Form most of the roof and superior portion of the side walls of cranium
2 **Temporal** bones Ⓞ	Contain mastoid sinuses, auditory meatus (ear canal), parts of ear, and the **styloid** Ⓞ1, **mastoid** Ⓞ2 and **zygomatic** Ⓞ3 **processes**	Form inferior sides, part of floor of the cranium
1 **Occipital** bone Ⓟ	Articulates with first vertebra; spinal cord passes through foramen magnum	Forms posterior portion and part of floor of the cranium
1 **Ethmoid** bone Ⓠ	Contains some paranasal sinuses, superior nasal conchae	Forms part of cranial floor, eye orbits, nasal septum, nasal cavity
1 **Sphenoid** bone Ⓡ	Articulates with all cranial bones; contains sphenoid sinus	Holds all cranial bones together; helps form eye orbit
Hyoid bone Ⓢ	U-shaped bone	Attaches to tongue

COLORING INSTRUCTIONS

Color each bone (or bone feature) and its name at the same time, using the same color.

1. As you read about the different bones, color them in both the anterior (top) and lateral (bottom) views.

2. Note that sometimes only one example of a bone (e.g., the maxillae) is labeled. Make sure you color both, if applicable.

3. Use dark colors to outline the cranial sutures (Ⓚ to Ⓝ).

4. If you wish, you can use darker versions of the same color to identify labeled bone characteristics. For example, you could color the temporal bones light blue, and the processes darker blue.

5. Color the blow-up drawings of the ethmoid Ⓠ and sphenoid Ⓡ bones.

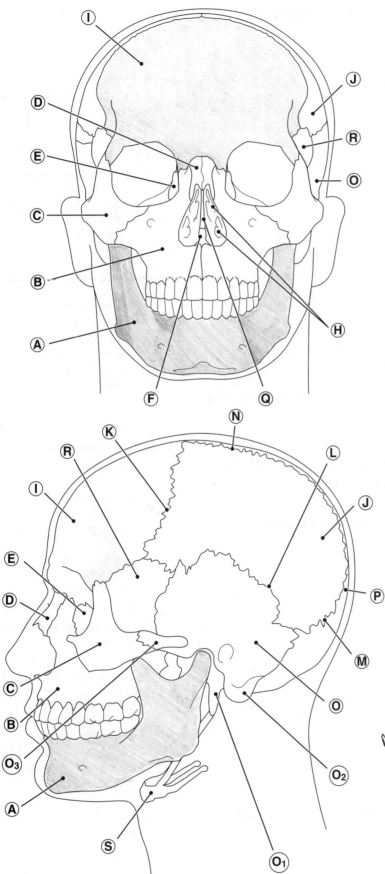

A. mandible
B. maxillae
C. zygomatic bone
D. nasal bone
E. lacrimal bone
F. vomer
G. palatine bone
H. inferior nasal conchae
I. frontal bone
J. parietal bone
K. coronal suture
L. squamous suture
M. lambdoid suture
N. sagittal suture
O. temporal bone
O_1. styloid process
O_2. mastoid process
O_3. zygomatic process
P. occipital bone
Q. ethmoid bone
R. sphenoid bone

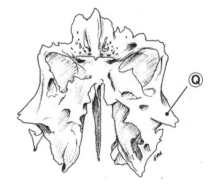

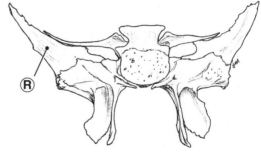

Coloring Exercise 3-7 ➤ The Vertebral Column

The Vertebral Column

Vertebrae are identified by region (C, T, L) and subsequently numbered from the most cephalic vertebra to the most caudal vertebra

- **Cervical vertebrae** (A)
  - Seven neck vertebrae, labelled C1 to C7
  - **Atlas** (C1) (B) supports the head
  - **Axis** (C2) (C) acts as a pivot to turn the head
- **Thoracic vertebrae** (D)
  - Twelve vertebrae located in chest, labelled T1 to T12
  - Ribs attach to long spinous processes (see top right figure)
- **Lumbar vertebrae** (E)
  - Five vertebrae located in the lower back, labelled L1 to L5
  - Very large and strong to support weight of torso
- **Sacral vertebrae** (F)
  - Five bones in child fuse to form one bone, the **sacrum** (F)
  - Sacrum forms the posterior part of the pelvis
- **Coccygeal vertebrae** (G)
  - Four or five bones in child fuse to form one bone, the **coccyx** (tail bone) (G)

Structure of a Vertebra

- **Intervertebral discs** (H) join together the **bodies** (I) of adjacent vertebrae
- The spinal cord passes through the **vertebral foramen** (J)
- Spinal nerves leave spinal cord through **intervertebral foramina** (K)
- The dorsal **spinous process** (L) and lateral **transverse processes** (M) of each vertebra are sites of muscle attachment
- The top right figures shows vertebra T6 in more detail.

Abnormal Curvatures

- **Kyphosis** (N): excessive thoracic curve
- **Lordosis** (O): excessive lumbar curve
- **Scoliosis** (P): abnormal lateral curvature

COLORING INSTRUCTIONS

Color each bone (or bone feature) and its name at the same time, using the same color. On the top figure:

1. Color the five types of vertebrae ((A), (D), (E), (F), and (G)) different *light* colors, but do not color C1 (B) or C2 (C). Write the name of each vertebra (e.g., T2) on or beside the bone. For the cervical vertebrae, use the spinous processes to guide you.

2. Use variants of the color used for the cervical vertebrae to color the atlas (B) and the axis (C).

COLORING INSTRUCTIONS

On the top right figures:

1. Color the parts of the vertebra (parts (H) to (L)). Use dark colors.

2. The parts of the vertebra are also labeled on the larger figure (top left). Color these parts on a few vertebrae.

COLORING INSTRUCTIONS

On the bottom figures:

1. Color the term describing the abnormal curvature and the corresponding vertebral column the same color ((N) to (P)).

2. Color the abnormal curve(s) with a darker version of the color.

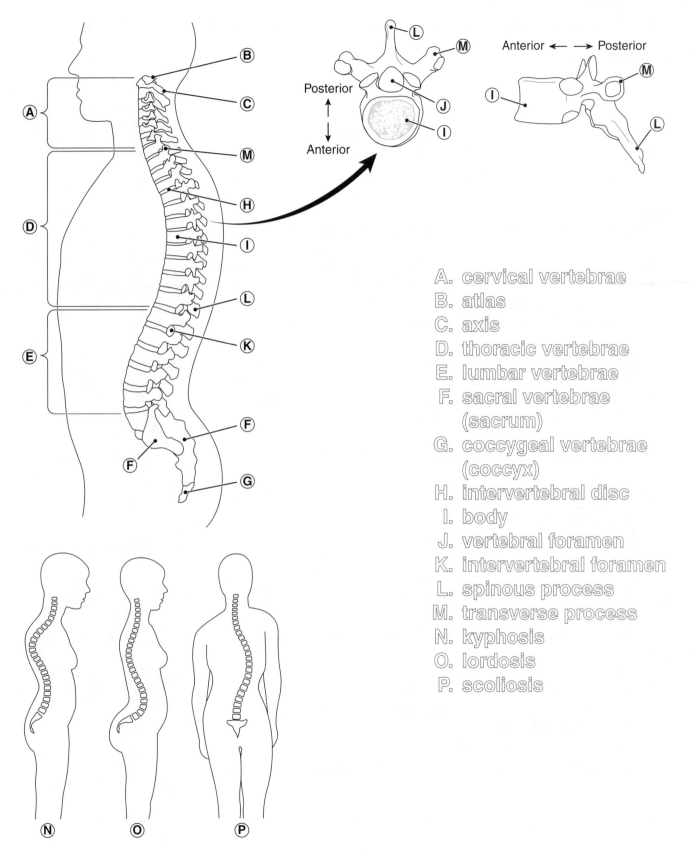

A. cervical vertebrae
B. atlas
C. axis
D. thoracic vertebrae
E. lumbar vertebrae
F. sacral vertebrae
   (sacrum)
G. coccygeal vertebrae
   (coccyx)
H. intervertebral disc
I. body
J. vertebral foramen
K. intervertebral foramen
L. spinous process
M. transverse process
N. kyphosis
O. lordosis
P. scoliosis

Coloring Exercise 3-8 ➤ The Thorax and Shoulder Girdle

The Thoracic Cage

- **Sternum** (A) + 12 pairs of ribs (and associated cartilage)
- Protects lungs, heart, kidneys, upper abdominal organs
- Supports bones of shoulder girdle and upper limbs
- Involved in respiration

Sternum (A)
- **Manubrium** (A1) joins with the clavicles at the **clavicular notch** (A2) and with the first pair of ribs
- Junction between manubrium and **body** (A3) can be felt as a ridge (the **sternal angle** (A4); identifies the second rib)
- Body joins the **costal cartilage** (B) of ribs two through seven
- **Xiphoid process** (A5) attached to some abdominal muscles

Ribs
- 12 pairs, attached to thoracic vertebrae 1–12
- **True ribs** (C) (pairs 1–7) attach directly to sternal body, via costal cartilages
- Some **false ribs** (D) (pairs 8–10) attach to the cartilage of the rib above
- Other false ribs (pairs 11 and 12—the **floating ribs** (E)) do not attach anteriorly
- **Intercostal space** (F): the space between ribs

The Shoulder Girdle

- Attaches upper limb to the axial skeleton
- Consists of the **clavicle** (G) and **scapula** (H)

Clavicle (Collarbone) (G)
- Articulates with sternum anteriorly, scapula laterally
- Sternoclavicular joint is the only bony connection between the upper limb (arm) and the axial skeleton
- S-shaped for increased strength; still site of frequent fractures

Scapula (Shoulder Blade) (H)
- Secured to axial skeleton by muscles
- Prominent ridge (**spine** (H1)) can be palpated
- Muscles attach to depressions (**supraspinous fossa** (H2), **infraspinous fossa** (H3)) and the **coracoid process** (H4)
- **Acromion** (H5) joins with the clavicle
- **Glenoid cavity** (H6) forms the shoulder joint with the **humerus** (I)

✐ COLORING INSTRUCTIONS

Color each bone (or bone feature) and its name at the same time, using the same color. On the top figure:

1. Color the sternum (A). You can use variants of the same color to distinguish between the manubrium (A1), body (A2), and xiphoid process (A3).
2. Color the costal cartilage (B) of all ribs.
3. Color the seven true ribs (C), false ribs (D), and floating ribs (E) using different light colors. Use closely related colors for the false and floating ribs, because floating ribs are a subtype of the false ribs.
4. Write the numbers of the rib pairs on each rib.
5. If you like, color some of the intercostal spaces (F) with a light color.

✐ COLORING INSTRUCTIONS

On the bottom figure:

1. Color the bones of the shoulder girdle ((G) and (H)) and the associated bones ((A) and (I)). Highlight the features of the scapula (H1) to (H6) using related, darker colors than the one used to color the scapula.

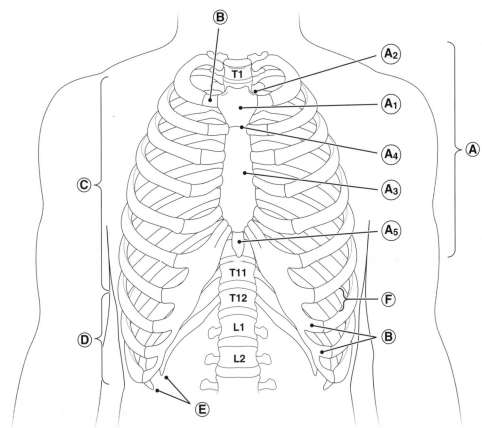

A. sternum
A₁. manubrium
A₂. clavicular notch
A₃. body
A₄. sternal notch
A₅. xiphoid process
B. costal cartilage
C. true ribs
D. false ribs
E. false (floating) ribs
F. intercostal space
G. clavicle
H. scapula
H₁. spine
H₂. supraspinous fossa
H₃. infraspinous fossa
H₄. coracoid process
H₅. acromion
H₆. glenoid cavity
I. humerus

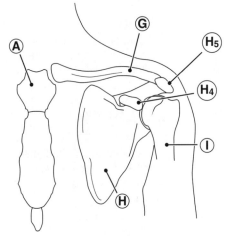

Anterior view

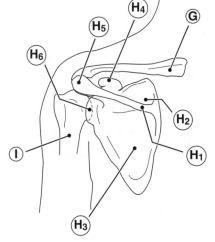

Posterior view

Coloring Exercise 3-9 ➤ The Upper Limb

The Arm

- The region between the shoulder and elbow
- Contains the **humerus** Ⓐ

Humerus Ⓐ
- **Head** Ⓐ1: helps form shoulder joint
- **Medial** Ⓐ2**/lateral** Ⓐ3 **epicondyles:** sites of attachment for forearm muscles
- Ulnar nerve passes over medial epicondyle; blows here produce tingling (hence, this area is called the funny bone)
- **Trochlea** (Ⓐ4 medial) and **capitulum** (Ⓐ5 lateral) help form elbow joint
- **Radial fossa** Ⓐ6 interacts with radius when elbow is bent
- **Olecranon fossa** Ⓐ7 interacts with ulna when elbow is straight

The Forearm

- The region between the elbow and wrist
- Consists of the **ulna** Ⓑ and **radius** Ⓒ
- Mnemonic: p.u. (*pinky* on *ulnar* side)

Ulna Ⓑ
- Medial bone (in anatomical position); longer than radius
- **Head** Ⓑ1 is at the wrist joint
- **Olecranon** Ⓑ2 forms elbow point
- **Trochlear notch** Ⓑ3 helps form elbow joint
- **Radial notch** Ⓑ4 interacts with radius
- Wrist ligaments attach to the **styloid process** Ⓑ5

Radius Ⓒ
- Lateral bone (in anatomical position)
- **Head** Ⓒ1 is at the elbow joint; **neck** Ⓒ2 is distal to the head
- Forearm muscles/wrist ligaments attach to **styloid process** Ⓒ3

Articulations

Shoulder joint Ⓓ: head of humerus articulates with glenoid cavity of scapula (ball and socket)

Elbow Joint Ⓔ
- Radius head interacts with humerus capitulum (hinge)
- Ulnar trochlear notch interacts with humerus trochlea (hinge)
- Radius head interacts with radial notch of ulna (pivot)

Wrist Joint Ⓕ
- Wrist ligaments bind styloid processes of ulna and radius
- Distal end of radius interacts with **carpal bones** Ⓖ
- Ulnar head interacts with ulnar notch of radius

Ulnar-radial Syndesmosis (fibrous joint): See Coloring Exercise 3-4

COLORING INSTRUCTIONS
Color each bone (or bone feature) and its name at the same time, using the same color. On the left figure:

1. Color the entire humerus Ⓐ light yellow.
2. Use darker versions of yellow and orange to highlight the different features of the humerus Ⓐ1 to Ⓐ7.

COLORING INSTRUCTIONS
On the right figure:

1. Color the radius Ⓑ light blue and the ulna Ⓒ light green.
2. Use darker versions of blue and green to highlight the different features of the radius Ⓑ1 to Ⓑ4 and ulna Ⓒ1 to Ⓒ3, respectively.

COLORING INSTRUCTIONS
On the small locator skeleton and on the right-hand figures:

1. Color the carpal bones Ⓖ.
2. Draw circles around the shoulder joint Ⓓ, elbow joint Ⓔ, and wrist joint Ⓕ using three different colors.
3. Note the bones involved in each joint.

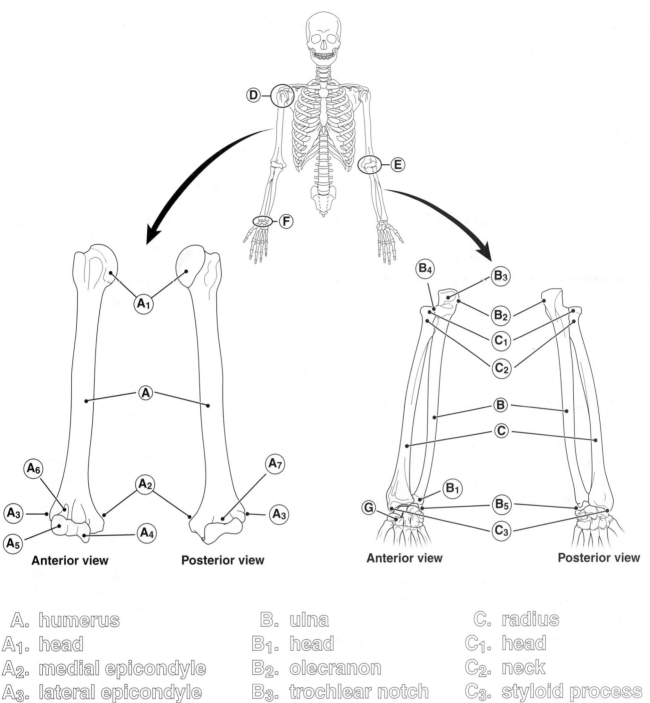

A. humerus
A₁. head
A₂. medial epicondyle
A₃. lateral epicondyle
A₄. trochlea
A₅. capitulum
A₆. radial fossa
A₇. olecranon fossa

B. ulna
B₁. head
B₂. olecranon
B₃. trochlear notch
B₄. radial notch
B₅. styloid process

C. radius
C₁. head
C₂. neck
C₃. styloid process

D. shoulder joint
E. elbow joint
F. wrist joint
G. carpal bones

Coloring Exercise 3-10 ➤ The Pelvis and Hip Joint

The Pelvis

- Two pelvic bones (ossa coxae, coxal bones)
- Each os coxae consists of three bones: **ilium** Ⓐ, **ischium** Ⓑ, and **pubis** Ⓒ that fuse together by age 23
- Ossa coxae joined anteriorly (**pubic symphysis** Ⓕ) and posteriorly (sacroiliac joint)
- All three bones form **acetabulum** Ⓓ (part of hip joint, see below)

Ilium Ⓐ

- Curved superior rim is the **iliac crest** Ⓐ1:
- **Anterior superior iliac spine** Ⓐ2: can be palpated (commonly described as the "hipbone")
- Articulates with **sacrum** Ⓔ

Ischium Ⓑ

- Largest, strongest pelvic bone
- **Ischial tuberosities** Ⓑ1: (commonly called the "sit bones") can be palpated below the buttock when in a seated position
- **Ischial spine** Ⓑ2: used as point of reference during childbirth

Pubis Ⓒ

- Two pubic bones join at **pubic symphysis** Ⓕ
- **Pubic arch** Ⓖ is wider in females than males
- Pubis and ischium form **obturator foramen** Ⓗ
  - 90%–95% of obturator foramen covered by membranes and muscles in living body

Hip Joint

- Strongest joint in the body (ball and socket)
- **Femoral head** Ⓘ sits in **acetabulum** Ⓓ of os coxae
- **Articular cartilage** Ⓙ protects both bone surfaces
- Very strong **joint capsule** Ⓚ supported by **ligaments** Ⓚ
- Extensive **synovial cavity** Ⓛ (also called a joint cavity) cushions joint

---

✎ COLORING INSTRUCTIONS

Color each bone (or bone feature) and its name at the same time, using the same color. Color both parts of the upper figure (anterior and posterior views) at the same time.

1. Use three different light colors to color the ilium Ⓐ, ischium Ⓑ, and pubis Ⓒ on each view.
2. Color the sacrum Ⓓ.
3. Use darker colors to highlight features of the ilium Ⓐ1 Ⓐ2 and ischium Ⓑ1 Ⓑ2.
4. Use a dark color to outline (anterior view) or color in (lateral view) portions of the os coxae contributing to the acetabulum Ⓓ.
5. Color the pubic symphysis Ⓕ and the obturator foramen Ⓗ.
6. Use a dark color to outline the pubic arch region Ⓖ.

✎ COLORING INSTRUCTIONS

Color the structures of the hip joint in the bottom figure.

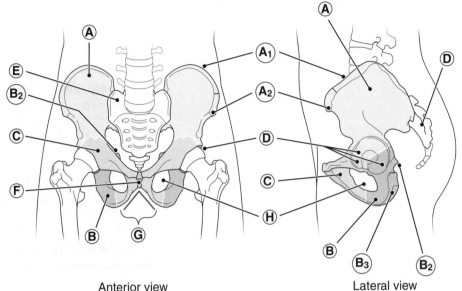

Anterior view   Lateral view

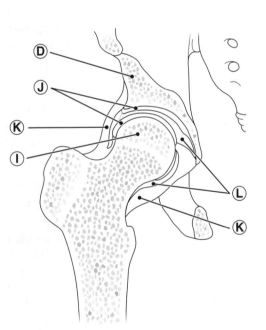

A. ilium
A₁. iliac crest
A₂. anterior superior
    iliac spine
B. ischium
B₁. ischial tuberosity
B₂. ischial spine
C. pubis
D. acetabulum
E. sacrum
F. pubic symphysis
G. pubic arch
H. obdurator foramen
I. femoral head
J. articular cartilage
K. joint capsule and
   ligaments
L. synovial cavity

Coloring Exercise 3-11 ➤ The Lower Limb

The Thigh

Region between the pelvis and knee

Femur (A)
- **Head** (A1) articulates with **pelvis** (B)
- **Neck** (A2): common site of fracture ("broken hip")
- Sites of thigh muscle attachment:
  - **Greater trochanter** (A3)
  - **Lesser trochanter** (A4)
  - **Linea aspera** (A5)
- **Medial** (A6) and **lateral** (A7) condyles articulate with tibia
- **Patellar surface** (A8) articulates with **patella** (C)
- **Medial epicondyle** (A9): attachment for knee ligaments

Patella (C)
- Enclosed within tendon of quadriceps femoris muscle
- Tracks between femoral condyles during knee movements

The Leg

- Region between the knee and ankle
- Contains the **tibia** (D) and the **fibula** (E) (LAteral fibuLA)

Tibia (D)
- Bears the weight of the entire body when standing
- **Lateral** (D1) and **medial** (D2) condyles articulate with femur
- **Anterior crest** (D3) can be palpated as the "shin bone"
- **Medial malleolus** (D4): inner prominence of ankle; articulates with **talus** (F)

Fibula (E)
- Not a weight-bearing bone; does not reach the knee
- **Head** (E1) interacts with tibial condyle
- **Lateral malleolus** (E2): outer prominence of ankle; articulates with talus

Articulations

- **Hip joint** (G): ball-and-socket joint between the femur head and the pelvis (see Coloring Exercise 3-10)
- **Knee joint** (H): hinge joint between the femur and tibia (Coloring Exercise 3-5)
- Tibiofibular joints
  - Tibia and fibula articulate **proximally** (I) and **distally** (J); these joints participate in rotating the lower leg (pivot joints)
  - Tibia and fibula bound longitudinally by an interosseous membrane (fibrous joint; not shown)

✍ COLORING INSTRUCTIONS

Color each bone (or bone feature) and its name at the same time, using the same color. On the top figure:

Color the six bones (A to F). Do not color any of the names of the bone features yet (for instance, (A1)).

✍ COLORING INSTRUCTIONS

Top right figure:

1. Color the entire femur (A) using light blue.
2. Use darker, related colors (blues and purples) to highlight the features of the femur ((A1) to (A9)).

✍ COLORING INSTRUCTIONS

Bottom figure:

1. Color the entire tibia (D) and fibula (E) using light colors (say, pink and light green).
2. Use darker, related colors (reds and darker greens) to highlight the features of the tibia ((D1) to (D4)) and the fibula ((E1) and (E2)).

✍ COLORING INSTRUCTIONS

Top left and bottom figures:

1. Circle the hip (G) and knee (H) joints on the left-hand figure (they are not labeled on the diagrams).
2. Circle the proximal (G) and distal (H) tibiofibular joints on both figures.

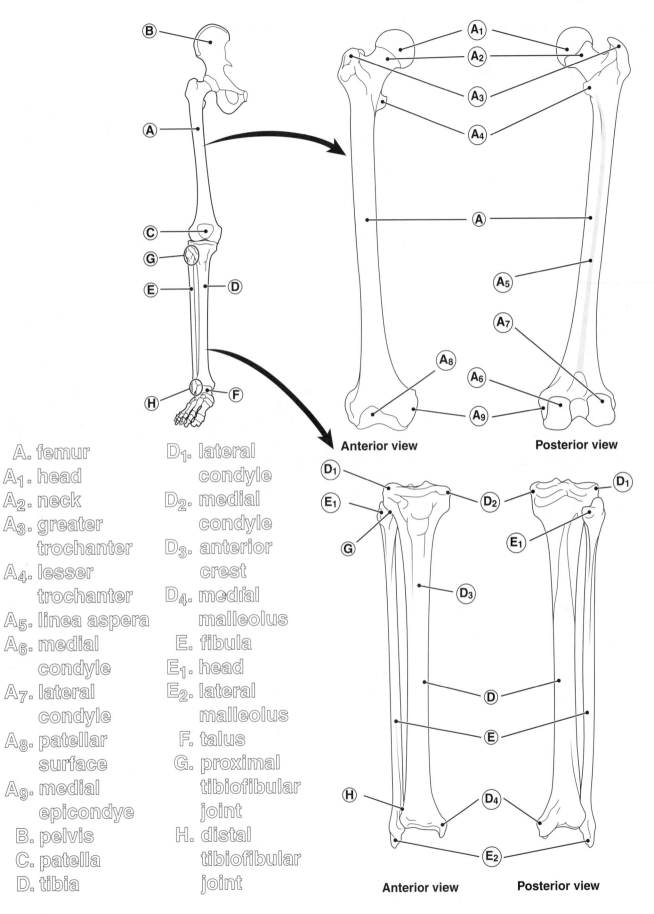

Anterior view   Posterior view

Anterior view   Posterior view

A. femur
A₁. head
A₂. neck
A₃. greater trochanter
A₄. lesser trochanter
A₅. linea aspera
A₆. medial condyle
A₇. lateral condyle
A₈. patellar surface
A₉. medial epicondye
B. pelvis
C. patella
D. tibia
D₁. lateral condyle
D₂. medial condyle
D₃. anterior crest
D₄. medial malleolus
E. fibula
E₁. head
E₂. lateral malleolus
F. talus
G. proximal tibiofibular joint
H. distal tibiofibular joint

Coloring Exercise 3-12 ➤ The Hand and Foot

Bones

Wrist and hand have the same basic plan as the ankle and foot

Wrist and Hand	Ankle and Foot
More mobile	Stronger, less mobile; arches of foot maintained by ligaments and tendons
Eight carpals in two rows (wrist)* • **scaphoid** Ⓐ • **lunate** Ⓑ • **triquetral** Ⓒ • **pisiform** Ⓓ • **trapezium** Ⓔ • **trapezoid** Ⓕ • **capitate** Ⓖ • **hamate** Ⓗ	Seven tarsals (ankle, foot) Anterior: • **cuboid** Ⓘ • three **cuneiforms** Ⓙ • **navicular** Ⓚ Posterior: • **talus** Ⓛ • **calcaneus** (heel) Ⓜ
Five **metacarpals** (palm) Ⓝ • Distal ends form knuckles • Numbered from 1 to 5, starting from the thumb side	Five **metatarsals** (instep) Ⓞ • Distal ends form ball of foot • Numbered from 1 to 5, starting from the great toe side
Fingers: three **phalanges (proximal** Ⓟ, **middle** Ⓠ, **distal** Ⓡ) Thumb: two phalanges (no middle phalanx)	Toes: three **phalanges (proximal** Ⓟ, **middle** Ⓠ, **distal** Ⓡ) Great toe: two phalanges (no middle phalanx)

* Mnemonic for the carpal bones: Stop Letting Those People Touch the Cadaver's Hand (Proximal, then Distal, Lateral to Medial) Edward Tanner, University of Alabama

Articulations

- Ankle: **talus** Ⓛ articulates with the **fibula** Ⓢ and **tibia** Ⓣ
- Wrist: three **carpals** Ⓐ, Ⓑ, and Ⓒ articulate with the **radius** Ⓤ and indirectly with the **ulna** Ⓥ
- Hand: condyloid joints between metacarpals and first finger phalanges; saddle joint between trapezium and first thumb phalanx; hinge joints between phalanges
- Foot: condyloid joints between metacarpals and toe phalanges; hinge joints between phalanges

✍🏻 **COLORING INSTRUCTIONS**

Color each bone (or bone feature) and its name at the same time, using the same color.

1. Color the diagrams of the hand (top) and foot (bottom) at the same time.
2. Color the carpal and tarsal bones (Ⓐ to Ⓜ) in related colors.
3. Color the metacarpal and metatarsal bones (Ⓝ and Ⓞ) in related colors.
4. Color the three types of phalanges (Ⓟ to Ⓡ) in related colors.
5. Color the other bones contributing to the ankle and wrist joints (Ⓢ to Ⓥ).

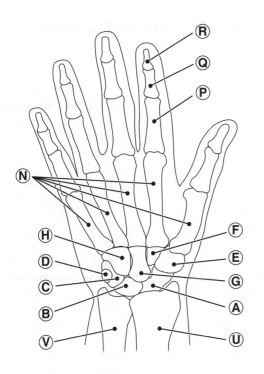

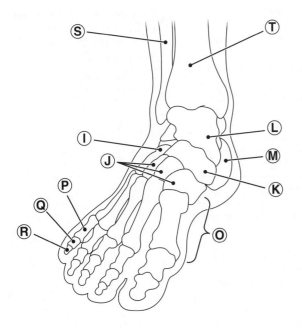

A. scaphoid
B. lunate
C. triquetral
D. pisiform
E. trapezium
F. trapezoid
G. capitate
H. hamate
I. cuboid
J. cuneiforms
K. navicular
L. talus
M. calcaneus
N. metacarpals
O. metatarsals
P. proximal phalanx
Q. middle phalanx
R. distal phalanx
S. fibula
T. tibia
U. radius
V. ulna

Coloring Exercise 3-13 ➤ Movements at Synovial Joints

Movement	Description	Examples
Flexion Ⓐ	Decreases angle between articulating bones in the sagittal plane	Touch chin to chest Raise arm in front of body[1] Bend upper limb at the elbow Move palm toward the forearm Move fingers toward the palm Raise thigh in front of body[2] Bend lower limb at knee joint
Extension Ⓑ	Increases angle between articulating bones in the sagittal plane (often returns to anatomical position) Hyperextension: movement continues beyond anatomical position	Raise head away from chest Lower arm in front of body Straighten arm at the elbow Move back of hand toward the forearm Move fingers away from the palm Swing thigh backwards[2] Straighten lower limb at the knee joint
Abduction Ⓒ	Movement away from the midline (frontal plane)	Move the arm laterally away from the body Move the thigh laterally away from the body[2] Bend hand towards thumb
Adduction Ⓓ	Movement toward the midline (frontal plane); restores anatomical position	Bring the arm laterally towards the body Move the thigh laterally toward the body[2] Bend hand away from thumb
Circumduction Ⓔ	Movement of the distal end of a bone in a circle	Circle the arm at the shoulder Circle the thigh at the hip[2]
Pronation Ⓕ	Palm faces posteriorly	Radioulnar joints only
Supination[3] Ⓖ	Palm faces anteriorly	Radioulnar joints only
Plantar flexion Ⓗ	Bend foot towards the plantar (bottom) surface	Ankle joint only: standing on toes
Dorsiflexion Ⓘ	Bend foot upwards	Ankle joint only: walk on heels
Inversion Ⓙ	Move feet to face each other	Ankle joint only: walk on lateral surface of feet
Eversion Ⓚ	Move feet to face away from each other	Ankle joint only: walk on medial surface of feet
Rotation Ⓛ	Bone revolves around its longitudinal axis	Turn head side to side

[1]Flexion at the shoulder joint is raising the arm.
[2]Actions illustrated for the shoulder joint also occur at the hip joint.
[3]Mnemonic: SUPinate to carry your SUPper.

Movements at the Shoulder (or Hip)

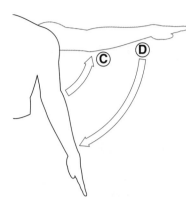 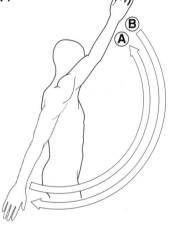 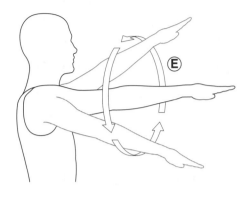

Movements of the Hand and Fingers

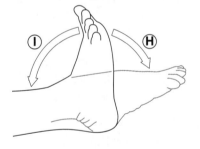 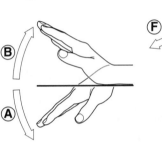 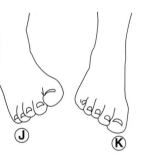 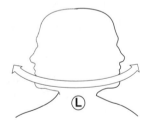

Movements of the Foot

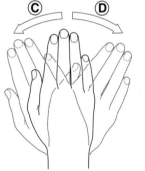

Movements of the Head

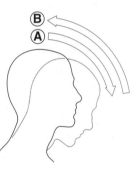

Movements at the Knee (or elbow)

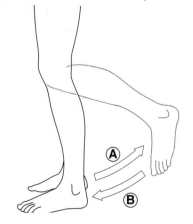

A. flexion
B. extension
C. abduction
D. adduction
E. circumduction
F. pronation

G. supination
H. plantar flexion
I. dorsiflexion
J. inversion
K. eversion
L. rotation

The Muscular System

Coloring Exercise 4-1 ➤ Muscle Tissue and Skeletal Muscle Anatomy

Muscle Tissue

- **Smooth muscle** Ⓐ: walls of hollow organs, blood vessels, and respiratory passages
- **Cardiac muscle** Ⓑ: wall of heart (see Coloring Exercise 8-6)
- **Skeletal muscle** Ⓒ: makes up muscles under voluntary control; moves bones and face, compresses abdominal organs
  - Several muscle cell precursors fuse to form a single muscle cell, containing multiple nuclei
- Muscle cells are also called fibers

Skeletal Muscle: Attachments to Bones

- **Tendons** Ⓓ attach skeletal muscle **body** Ⓔ to bones
- **Origin** Ⓕ: attachment to less moveable bone (e.g., **scapula** Ⓖ)
- **Insertion** Ⓗ: attachment to more moveable bone (e.g., **radius** Ⓘ)

Anatomy of a Skeletal Muscle

- Muscle enveloped by a membrane, the **epimysium** Ⓙ
  - The **tendon** Ⓓ is a continuation of the epimysium
- Skeletal muscle body divided into **fascicles** Ⓚ
  - Each fascicle surrounded by membrane; the **perimysium** Ⓛ
  - **Blood vessels** Ⓜ travel between fascicles
- Each fascicle made up of individual **muscle cells** Ⓒ
  - Each muscle cell surrounded by **endomysium** Ⓝ membrane
- Remember, you already colored a longitudinal view of skeletal muscle fibers in the top figure

---

✎ COLORING INSTRUCTIONS

Color each structure and its name at the same time, using the same color. On the top figure:

1. Color the nuclei black in each figure.
2. Color the muscle cells for each muscle type (Ⓐ to Ⓒ).

✎ COLORING INSTRUCTIONS

On the middle figure:

1. Color the bones (Ⓖ, Ⓘ), tendons Ⓓ, and the muscle body Ⓔ. Use light colors for the bones (Ⓖ, Ⓘ) and the muscle body.
2. Using two dark colors, draw circles at the origins Ⓕ and insertion Ⓗ of the muscle.

✎ COLORING INSTRUCTIONS

On the bottom figure:

1. Color the bone Ⓘ, tendon Ⓓ, and epimysium Ⓙ.
2. Color the perimysium Ⓛ around the extruded fascicle and in the cross section.
3. Color the fascicle Ⓚ that is labeled in the cross section, and one additional fascicle.
4. Color the endomysium Ⓝ around the extruded muscle fiber. Outline some muscle fibers in the cross-section with the same color, because the endomysium surrounds all fibers.
5. Color the ends of some muscle fibers Ⓒ and the blood vessels Ⓜ.

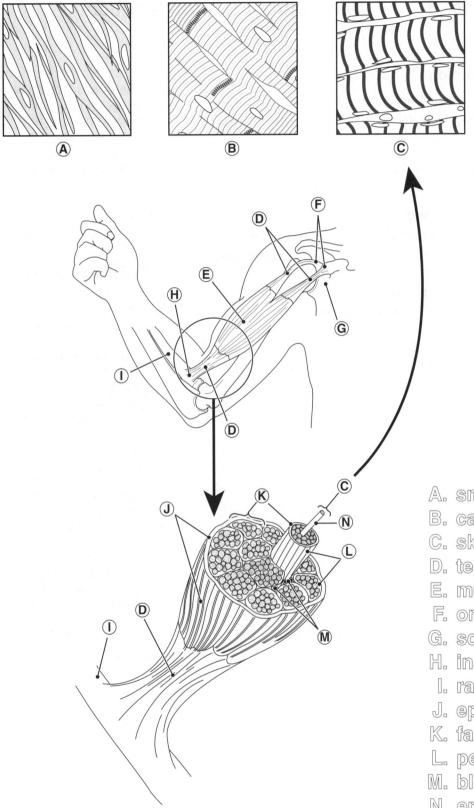

A. smooth muscle cells
B. cardiac muscle cells
C. skeletal muscle cells
D. tendon
E. muscle body
F. origin
G. scapula
H. insertion
 I. radius
J. epimysium
K. fasicle
L. perimysium
M. blood vessel
N. endomysium

Coloring Exercise 4-2 ➤ The Neuromuscular Junction

The Neuromuscular Junction

- Consists of a **muscle cell** (A) and **motor neuron** (B)
- Each muscle cell contains multiple **nuclei** (C)

Components of a Muscle Cell

- Muscle cell organized into **sarcomeres** (D)
- Each sarcomere contains **actin** (thin) (E) and **myosin** (thick) (F) filaments

Events at the Neuromuscular Junction

- **Action potential** (G) arrives at **axon branches** (B1) of a **motor neuron** (B)
- **Synaptic vesicles** (H) containing stored neurotransmitters (**acetylcholine**, (I)) fuse with the neuron membrane
- Acetylcholine released into the **synaptic cleft** (J)
- Acetylcholine binds **receptor** (K) in the **motor end plate** (L) (muscle cell membrane)
- Bound receptor creates action potential in muscle cell
- **Mitochondria** (M) make some neurotransmitters and provide ATP

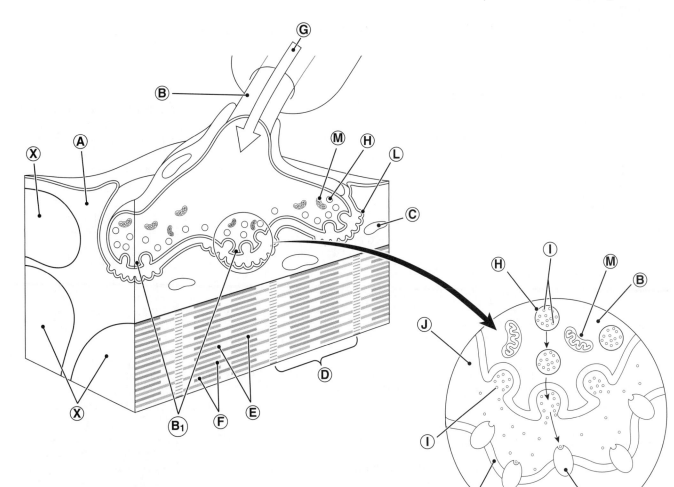

A. muscle cell
B. motor neuron
B$_1$. axon branches
C. nucleus
D. sarcomere
E. actin
F. myosin

G. action potential
H. synaptic vesicle
I. acetylcholine
J. synaptic cleft
K. receptor
L. motor end plate
M. mitochondria

Coloring Exercise 4-3 ➤ Muscle Contraction

The Sliding Filament Mechanism

- Remember that each muscle fiber is organized in **sarcomeres** Ⓐ
- Each sarcomere contains overlapping filaments of
  - **Myosin** Ⓑ: long filamentous protein with globular head
  - **Actin** Ⓒ: globular protein linked together in long strands; each actin has a **binding site** Ⓓ for myosin
- During muscle contraction, sarcomeres SHORTEN
  - The length of myosin and actin filaments does not change
  - The overlap between thick and thin filaments increases; filaments "slide over" each other
  - As sarcomeres shorten, the muscle shortens
- Sliding filament mechanism includes three stages
  - **Attachment** Ⓔ: **myosin** Ⓑ binds specific **binding sites** Ⓓ on the **actin** Ⓒ, forming a cross-bridge
  - **Power Stroke** Ⓕ: Myosin pulls on actin, shortening the sarcomere (and thus the muscle)
  - **Release/Reattachment** Ⓖ: Myosin head detaches (step requires fresh ATP molecule), binds further along the actin molecule
  - Cycle repeats

Calcium and Muscle Contraction

- The sliding filament mechanism only occurs if **calcium** Ⓗ is present
- Calcium is present in the muscle cell following an action potential in the motor end plate
- If calcium is absent;
  - **Tropomyosin** Ⓘ covers the **binding sites** Ⓓ
  - The three-part **troponin complex** Ⓙ keeps tropomyosin in place
- If calcium is present:
  - Calcium binds troponin
  - Troponin lets tropomyosin move away from binding sites on actin
  - Myosin heads can bind actin
  - Muscle contraction occurs

✍ **COLORING INSTRUCTIONS**

Color each structure and its name at the same time, using the same color. On the top figure:

1. Use the same colors for structures Ⓐ to Ⓒ as you used in the previous Coloring Exercise.
2. Color the bracket representing the sarcomere Ⓐ.
3. For the top diagram, color the bracket representing the name of the stage Ⓔ.
4. Lightly color the myosin Ⓑ and actin Ⓒ molecules. Color the actin binding sites Ⓓ using a dark color.
5. Repeat steps 3 and 4 for the other two diagrams, representing stages Ⓕ and Ⓖ.
6. After coloring all three diagrams, note that the overlap between thick and thin filaments increases. This results in shortening of both the sarcomere and the muscle.
7. Note that the myosin heads reattach to a different site on the actin molecules.

✍ **COLORING INSTRUCTIONS**

On the bottom figure:

1. Color all of the components in the top diagram, when calcium is not present.
2. Color all of the components in the bottom diagram, when calcium is present.

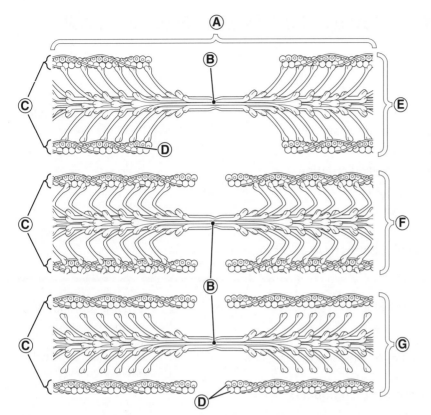

A. sarcomere
B. myosin
C. actin
D. binding site
E. attachment
F. power stroke
G. release/reattachment
H. calcium
 I. tropomyosin
J. troponin complex

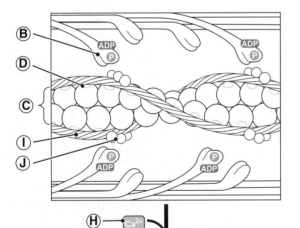

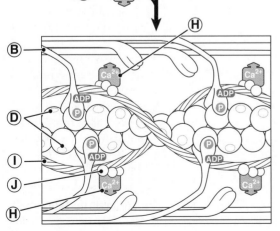

Coloring Exercise 4-4 ➤ Energy for Working Muscles: ATP

Where do Muscles Obtain ATP?

Creatine phosphate Ⓑ
- Very rapid **ATP** Ⓐ production; no oxygen or glucose required
- Muscles contain small store of creatine phosphate
- Creatine phosphate loses phosphate group, creating **creatine** Ⓒ
- **ADP** Ⓓ accepts phosphate group, resulting in **ATP** Ⓐ
- Creatine phosphate stores increased by exercise, dietary supplementation

Anaerobic metabolism Ⓔ
- **Glucose** Ⓕ rapidly converted into small amount of **ATP** Ⓐ (2–3 molecules); no **oxygen** Ⓖ required
- **Lactic acid** Ⓗ produced as byproduct
- Glucose can come from blood or (more frequently) from **glycogen** Ⓘ breakdown

Aerobic metabolism Ⓙ
- Glucose slowly converted into large amount of ATP (over 30 molecules); oxygen required
- Oxygen is stored within muscle cells attached to **myoglobin** Ⓚ
- Other energy sources (amino acids, fatty acids) can also be used

Why do Muscles Need ATP?

- **Power stroke** Ⓛ: movement of the myosin head that brings actin filaments closer together
- **Myosin head detachment** Ⓜ: no ATP results in rigor mortis: myosin heads stay attached, muscle cannot relax
- **Calcium reuptake** Ⓝ
  - Calcium reuptake into endoplasmic reticulum necessary for muscle relaxation
  - Occurs by active transport

✍ **COLORING INSTRUCTIONS**

Color each structure and its name at the same time, using the same color. On the top figure:

1. Color the terms ADP, creatine phosphate, and creatine.
2. Color the ATP molecule of this diagram bright green.

✍ **COLORING INSTRUCTIONS**

1. Color the glycogen Ⓘ and glucose Ⓔ molecules using related colors. Note that glycogen is actually made up of many glucose molecules.
2. Color the anaerobic arrow Ⓔ and the weightlifter with the same color.
3. Color the adjacent oxygen molecule Ⓖ. Draw a black X over it to indicate that oxygen is not used.
4. Color the two ATP molecules Ⓐ and the lactic acid Ⓗ.

✍ **COLORING INSTRUCTIONS**

1. Color the aerobic arrow Ⓙ and the cross-country skier with the same color.
2. Color the adjacent oxygen molecules Ⓖ and myoglobin Ⓚ.
3. Color the ATP molecules Ⓐ. Not all of the ATPs are shown—one glucose molecule can produce over 30 ATPs.

✍ **COLORING INSTRUCTIONS**

Color the terms Ⓛ to Ⓝ and the accompanying cartoons.

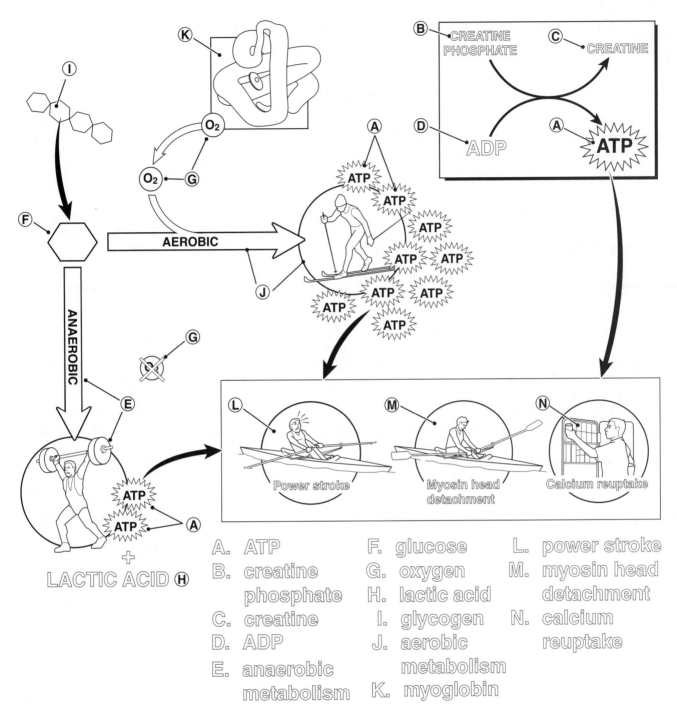

A. ATP
B. creatine phosphate
C. creatine
D. ADP
E. anaerobic metabolism
F. glucose
G. oxygen
H. lactic acid
I. glycogen
J. aerobic metabolism
K. myoglobin
L. power stroke
M. myosin head detachment
N. calcium reuptake

Coloring Exercise 4-5 ➤ Muscles in Action

Muscles Work Together to Produce a Given Action

- **Prime mover** (A): accomplishes movement
- **Antagonist** (B): produces opposite movement
  - Must relax to permit prime mover contraction
- **Synergist** (C): assists prime mover by providing additional force or by stabilizing joint
- Synergists and prime movers are also called agonists

An Example: Movements of the Forearm

- Bend your arm at a right angle; hold a weight in your hand
- During each action, use your other hand to feel muscles contract and relax
- Flexion (figure on left)
  - Bring your hand towards your shoulder
  - Prime mover: **brachialis** (D) (front of upper arm) contracts
  - Antagonist: **triceps brachii** (E) (back of upper arm) relaxes
  - Synergist: **brachioradialis** (F) (lower arm) contracts
- Extension (figure on right)
  - Slowly lower your hand
  - Prime mover: triceps brachii contracts (the biceps brachii [not shown] is also a prime mover)
  - Antagonists: brachialis and brachioradialis relax

Flexion

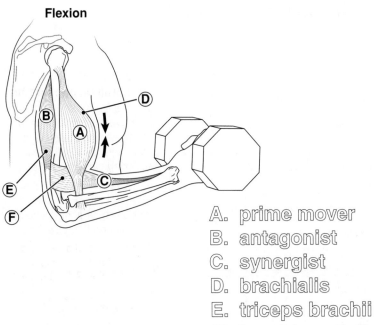

Extension

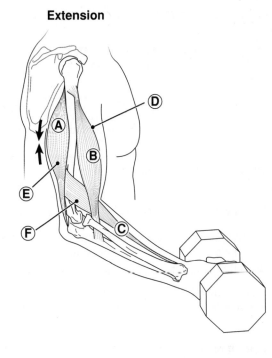

A. prime mover
B. antagonist
C. synergist
D. brachialis
E. triceps brachii
F. brachioradialis

Coloring Exercise 4-6 ➤ Muscles of the Head

Name	Origin	Insertion	Action
Frontalis Ⓐ	**Epicranial aponeurosis** (tendon Ⓟ)	Eyebrow skin	Raises eyebrows
Obicularis oculi Ⓑ	Frontal bone, maxilla (eye orbit)	Skin, muscle encircling eye	Closes eye
Nasalis Ⓒ	Maxilla	Bridge of nose	Moves nose
Levator palpebrae superioris (not shown)	Sphenoid bone (roof of eye orbit)	Upper eyelid skin	Opens eye
Quadratus labii superioris Ⓓ	Maxilla	Obicularis oris; skin at lip corners	Elevates upper lip
Zygomaticus Ⓔ	Zygomatic bone	Skin, muscle at lip corners	Raises corner(s) of mouth
Obicularis oris Ⓕ	Muscles encircling mouth	Skin at mouth corners	Closes lips (kissing), shapes lips (speech)
Quadratus labii inferioris Ⓖ	Mandible	Lower lip skin	Depresses lower lip
Mentalis Ⓗ	Mandible	Chin skin	Elevates, protrudes lower lip (pouting)
Triangularis Ⓘ (Depressor anguli oris)	Mandible	Mouth (angle)	Opens mouth
Buccinator Ⓙ	Maxilla, mandible	Obicularis oris	Flattens cheek (eating, whistling, wind instruments)
Digastricus Ⓚ	Mandible, temporal bone	Hyoid bone (via tendon)	Opens jaw
Masseter Ⓛ	Temporal bone	Mandible	Closes jaw
Sternocleido-mastoid Ⓜ	Sternum, clavicle	Temporal bone (mastoid process)	Together: flexes head Separately: rotates head
Temporalis Ⓝ	Temporal bone	Mandible	Closes jaw
Trapezius Ⓞ: see Coloring Exercise 4-7			

✎ **COLORING INSTRUCTIONS**

Color each muscle and its name at the same time, using the same color. Color the lateral (top) and frontal (bottom) views together.

1. Review the skull bones in Coloring Exercise 3-6 before beginning this Coloring Exercise.
2. As you read about each muscle, try to palpate the insertion and origin.
3. Use the muscle to perform the action. Use your fingers to feel the muscle contract.
4. Color the muscle on the diagram(s).
5. Use a very light color for Ⓟ, because this structure is not a muscle.

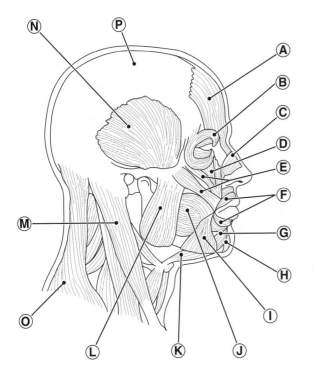

A. frontalis
B. obicularis oculi
C. nasalis
D. quadratus labii superioris
E. zygomaticus
F. obicularis oris
G. quadratus labii inferioris
H. mentalis
I. triangularis
J. buccinator
K. digastricus
L. masseter
M. sternoocleidomastoid
N. temporalis
O. trapezius
P. epicranial aponeurosis

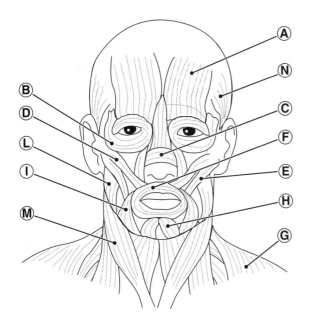

Coloring Exercise 4-7 ➤ Muscles of the Torso

Abdominal Muscles

Name	Origin	Insertion	Action
Rectus abdominus Ⓐ	Pubis	Xiphoid process (sternum), ribs	Flexes spinal column, compresses abdomen
External oblique Ⓑ	Inferior eight ribs	Ilium, **linea alba** Ⓒ	Both: flex spinal column, compress abdomen One: rotate, laterally flex spinal column
Internal oblique Ⓓ	Iliac crest	Inferior ribs, linea alba	Same as external obliques
Transverse abdominis Ⓔ	Iliac crest, inferior ribs	Xyxoid process, linea alba, pubis	Compresses abdomen
Abdominal aponeurosis Ⓕ (tendon)			

Muscles of the Perineum

Name	Origin	Insertion	Action
Transverse perineus Ⓖ	**Ischial tuberosity** Ⓗ	Perineal tissues (**vagina** Ⓘ)	Stabilizes perineum
Levator ani Ⓙ	Pubis, ischial spine	**Coccyx** Ⓚ, **urethra** Ⓛ, rectum, perineum	Aids defecation; stabilizes perineum
External anal sphincter Ⓜ	Anococcygeal ligament, coccyx	Perineal tissues	Closes **anus** Ⓝ
Ischiocavernosus Ⓞ	Ischial tuberosity, pubis	**Clitoris** Ⓟ, penis	Maintains clitoral or penile erection
Bulbocavernosus Ⓠ	Perineal tissues	Clitoris, penis, other perineal tissues	Maintains clitoral or penile erection; aids in urination, ejaculation; constricts vagina
Coccygeus Ⓡ	Ischium	Coccyx, lower sacrum	Stabilizes perineum; pulls coccyx forward during defecation, childbirth
Obturator Ⓢ	Obturator foramen	Femur (greater trochanter)	Rotates thigh
Gluteus maximus Ⓣ	See Coloring Exercise 4-9		

✏️ **COLORING INSTRUCTIONS**

Color each muscle and its name at the same time, using the same color. On the top figure:

1. As you read about each muscle, try to palpate the insertion and origin.
2. Use the muscle to perform the action. Use your fingers to feel the muscle contract.
3. Color the muscle on the diagram.
4. Color the tendons; the linea alba Ⓒ and the abdominal aponeurosis Ⓕ.

✏️ **COLORING INSTRUCTIONS**

On the bottom figure:

1. As you read about each muscle, use the muscle to perform the action (where possible).
2. Color the muscle on the diagram.
3. Use very light colors for structures that are not muscles (Ⓗ, Ⓘ, Ⓚ, Ⓛ, Ⓟ).

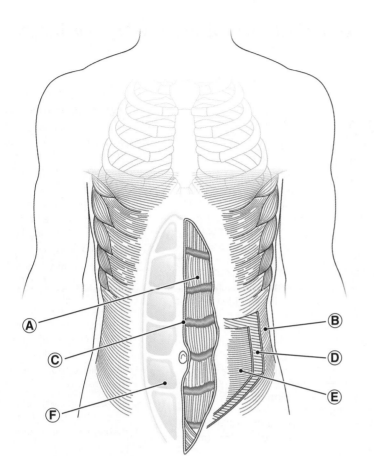

A. rectus abdominis
B. external oblique
C. linea alba
D. internal oblique
E. transverse abdominis
F. abdominal aponeurosis
G. transverse perineus
H. ischial tuberosity
I. vagina
J. levator ani
K. coccyx
L. urethra
M. external anal sphincter
N. anus
O. ischiocavernosus
P. clitoris
Q. bulbocavernosus
R. coccygeus
S. obturator
T. gluteus maximus

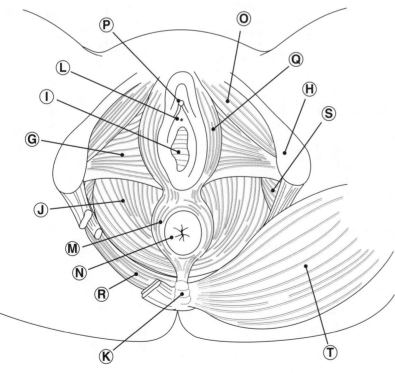

Coloring Exercise 4-8 ➤ Muscles that Move the Upper Limb

Name	Origin	Insertion	Action
Trapezius (A)	Occipital bone, vertebrae (C7, thoracic)	Clavicle, scapula (acromion, spine)	Extends head; raises shoulder and pulls it posteriorly; stabilizes and moves scapula
Latissimus dorsi (B)	Vertebrae, sacrum, ilium, ribs	Humerus	Extends and adducts arm (behind back)
Pectoralis major (C)	Clavicle, sternum, cartilage of ribs 2–6	Humerus	Flexes and adducts arm (across chest); pulls shoulder forward and down
Serratus anterior (D)	Superior ribs	Scapula	Moves scapula forward; aids in punching, reaching
Teres major (E)	Scapula	Humerus	Extends arm
Teres minor (F)	Scapula	Humerus	Extends, adducts arm; part of rotator cuff
Deltoid (G)	Clavicle, scapula	Humerus	Abducts arm
Biceps brachii (H)	Scapula	Proximal radius	Flexes forearm, supinates hand
Brachioradialis (I)	Humerus	Radius	Flexes forearm
Brachialis (J)	Humerus	Ulna	Flexes forearm
Triceps brachii (K)	Scapula, humerus	Ulnar olecranon	Extends forearm
Extensor carpi radialis longus (L)	Humerus	2nd metacarpal	Extends, abducts hand
Flexor carpi radialis (M)	Humerus	2nd and 3rd metacarpals	Flexes, abducts hand
Flexor carpi ulnaris (N)	Humerus, ulna	5th metacarpal	Flexes, adducts hand
Extensor carpi ulnaris (O)	Humerus, posterior ulna	5th metacarpal	Extends, adducts hand
Flexor digitorum superficialis (P)	Humerus, ulna, radius	Middle phalanx, each finger	Flexes fingers
Extensor digitorum (Q)	Humerus	Distal and medial phalanges, each finger	Extends fingers

✍ **COLORING INSTRUCTIONS**

Color each muscle and its name at the same time, using the same color. Color the anterior and posterior views together.

1. Review the bones of the shoulder girdle and upper limb in Coloring Exercises 3-8 and 3-9.

2. Review the movements of the upper limb in Coloring Exercise 3-13. Remember that movements at the shoulder joint move the arm and movements at the elbow joint move the forearm.

3. As you read about each muscle, try to palpate the insertion and origin.

4. Use the muscle to perform the action. Use your fingers to feel the muscle contract.

5. Color the muscle on the diagram.

Anterior view

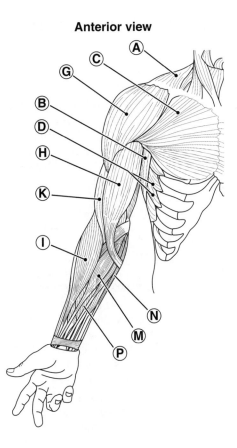

A. trapezius
B. latissimus dorsi
C. pectoralis major
D. serratus anterior
E. teres major
F. teres minor
G. deltoid
H. biceps brachii
 I. brachioradialis
J. triceps brachii
K. brachialis
L. extensor carpi
   radialis longus
M. flexor carpi
   radialis
N. flexor carpi
   ulnaris
O. extensor carpi
   ulnaris
P. flexor digitorum
   superficialis
Q. extensor digitorum

Posterior view

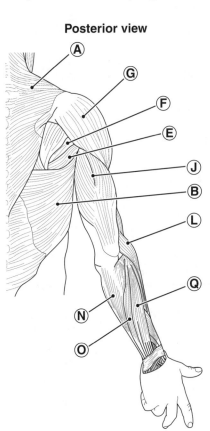

Coloring Exercise 4-9 ➤ Muscles that Move the Lower Limb

Name	Origin	Insertion	Action
Iliopsoas Ⓐ	Ilium, lumbar vertebrae	Femur (lesser trochanter)	Flexes hip
Sartorius Ⓑ	Iliac spine	Tibia body	Flexes thigh, leg
Quadriceps Femoris Group:			
Rectus femoris Ⓒ	Iliac spine	Patella, then tibia	Extends leg; flexes hip
Vastus lateralis Ⓓ	Femur (greater trochanter, linea aspera)	Patella, then tibia	Extends leg
Vastus medialis Ⓔ	Femur (greater trochanter, linea aspera)	Patella, then tibia	Extends leg
Vastus intermedius	Femur	Patella, then tibia	Extends leg
Adductor longus Ⓕ	Pubic crest and symphysis	Femur (linea aspera)	Adducts thigh
Gracilis Ⓖ	Pubis	Tibia	Adducts thigh; flexes leg
Adductor magnus Ⓗ	Pubis, ischium	Femur (linea aspera)	Adducts thigh
Gluteus medius Ⓘ	Ilium	Femur (greater trochanter)	
Gluteus maximus Ⓙ	Iliac crest, sacrum, coccyx	Iliotibial tract, femur (linea aspera)	
Hamstring Group:			
Biceps femoris Ⓚ	Ischial tuberosity, linea aspera of femur	Fibula (head) and tibia (lateral condyle)	Flexes leg; extends hip
Semitendinosus Ⓛ	Ischial tuberosity	Proximal tibia	Flexes leg; extends hip
Semimembranosus Ⓜ	Ischial tuberosity	Tibia (medial condyle)	Flexes leg; extends hip
Peroneus longus Ⓝ	Fibula, tibia (lateral condyle)	First tarsal and first metatarsal of foot	Everts foot
Tibialis anterior Ⓞ	Tibia: lateral condyle/body	1st tarsal, 1st metatarsal	Dorsiflexes, inverts foot
Gastrocnemius Ⓟ	femur: lateral, medial condyles	Calcaneus (via Achilles tendon)	Plantar flexes foot
Soleus Ⓠ	Fibula (head) and proximal tibia	Calcaneus (via Achilles tendon)	Plantar flexes foot
Extensor digitorum longus Ⓡ	Tibia	Distal phalanges, 2nd to 5th toes	Extends toes
Flexor digitorum longus Ⓢ	Posterior tibia	Distal phalanges, 2nd to 5th toes	Flexes toes
Iliotibial tract (tendon) Ⓣ	Gluteus maximus	Tibia (lateral condyle)	Tendon

COLORING INSTRUCTIONS

Color each muscle and its name at the same time, using the same color. Color the anterior and posterior views together.

1. Review the bones of the pelvis and lower limb in Coloring Exercises 3-10 and 3-11.

2. Review the movements of the lower limb in Coloring Exercise 3-13. Remember that movements at the hip joint move the thigh, and movements at the knee joint move the leg (tibia/fibula).

3. Label some of the bone features that you see in this diagram, such as the patella, tibia, and calcaneus.

4. As you read about each muscle, try to palpate the insertion and origin.

5. Use the muscle to perform the action. Use your fingers to feel the muscle contract.

6. Color the muscle on the diagram. Color the iliotibial tract Ⓣ a very light color, because it is not a muscle.

Anterior view

Posterior view

A. iliopsoas
B. sartorius
C. rectus femoris
D. vastus lateralis
E. vastus medialis
F. adductor longus
G. gracilis
H. adductor magnus
I. gluteus medius
J. gluteus maximus
K. biceps femoris
L. semitendinosus
M. semimembranosus
N. peroneus longus
O. tibialis anterior
P. gastrocnemius
Q. soleus
R. extensor digitorum longus
S. flexor digitorum longus
T. iliotibial tract

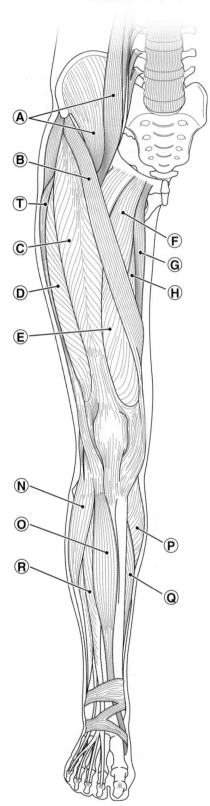

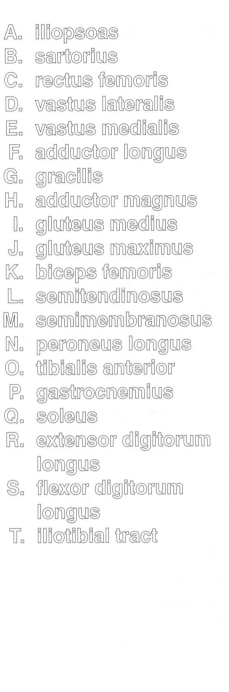

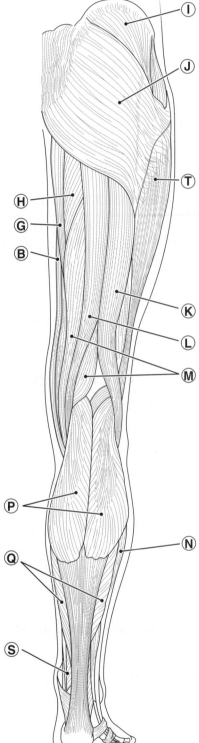

Coloring Exercise 4-10 ➤ Skeletal Muscle Review (Part 1)

Stabilizers

- Scapula (stabilization and movement): trapezius, serratus anterior
- Shoulder joint: rotator cuff (supraspinatus, infraspinatus, teres minor, subscapularis)
- Perineum: transverse perineus, levator ani, coccygeus
- Abdominal organs: transverse abdominus, rectus abdominus, internal and external obliques

Movements at the Shoulder Joint

- The humerus moves relative to the pectoral girdle
- Flexion: pectoralis major, anterior deltoid (both prime movers)
- Extension: latissimus dorsi (prime mover) teres major, teres minor, posterior deltoid
- Abduction: deltoid
- Adduction: latissimus dorsi (prime mover) pectoralis major, teres minor
- Rotation: pectoralis major, teres major, latissimus dorsi

Movements at the Elbow Joint

- The ulna/radius move relative to the humerus
- Flexion: brachialis (prime mover) biceps brachii, brachioradialis
- Extension: triceps brachii

Movements at the Wrist Joint

- The hand moves relative to the ulna/radius
- Flexion: flexor carpi radialis, flexor carpi ulnaris
- Extension: extensor carpi radialis longus
- Abduction: flexor carpi radialis, extensor carpi radialis longus
- Adduction: flexor carpi ulnaris

Movements of the Fingers

- Flexion: flexor digitorum superficialis
- Extension: extensor digitorum

✎ COLORING INSTRUCTIONS

Coloring Exercises 4-10 and 4-11 categorize muscles by the actions they produce. The accompanying figures only show the superficial muscles. Some of the muscles discussed in the narrative are deep muscles and thus are not illustrated.

1. Review the muscles involved in each action.
2. Write the names of the muscles in the blanks. The answers are in Appendix I at the back of the book.

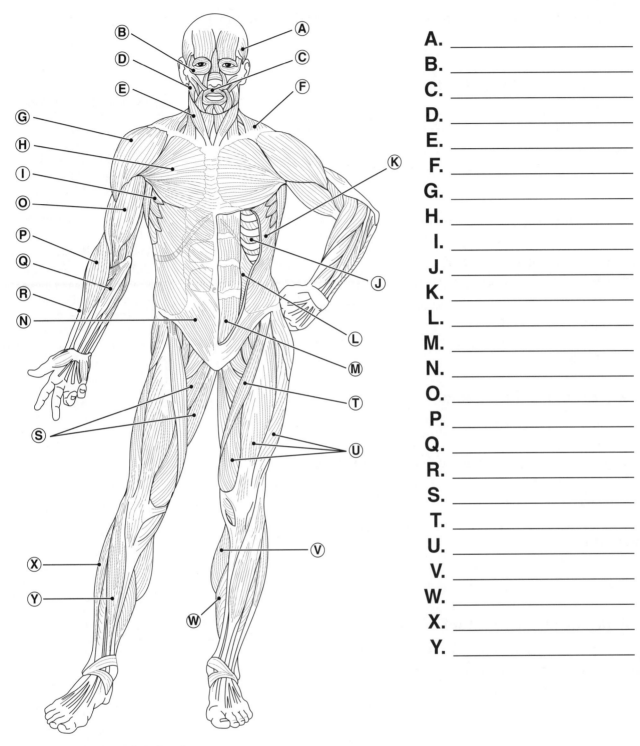

Anterior view

A. _____

B. _____

C. _____

D. _____

E. _____

F. _____

G. _____

H. _____

I. _____

J. _____

K. _____

L. _____

M. _____

N. _____

O. _____

P. _____

Q. _____

R. _____

S. _____

T. _____

U. _____

V. _____

W. _____

X. _____

Y. _____

Coloring Exercise 4-11 ➤ Skeletal Muscle Review (Part 2)

Movements at the Thigh Joint

- The femur moves relative to the pelvis
- Flexion: iliopsoas (prime mover), sartorius (weak flexor; used for sitting cross-legged), rectus femoris
- Extension: gluteus maximus (especially when climbing or jumping), hamstring group
- Abduction: gluteus medius
- Adduction: adductor longus, adductor magnus, gracilis

Movements at the Knee Joint

- The tibia/fibula move relative to the femur
- Flexion: hamstring group (biceps femoris, semimembranosus, semitendinosus), gracilis, sartorius (weak)
- Extension: quadriceps group (rectus femoris, vastus medialis, vastus lateralis, vastus intermedius)

Movements at the Ankle Joint

- The foot moves relative to the tibia/fibula
- Dorsiflexion: tibialis anterior
- Plantar flexion: gastrocnemius (prime mover), soleus
- Inversion: tibialis anterior
- Eversion: peroneus longus

Movements of the Toes

- Flexion: flexor digitorum groups
- Extension: extensor digitorum groups

Maintenance of Body Posture

- Gluteus maximus: supports upright posture
- Gluteus medius: stabilizes pelvis during walking
- Iliopsoas: prevents upper body from falling backward when standing erect

---

COLORING INSTRUCTIONS

Coloring Exercises 4-10 and 4-11 categorize muscles by the actions they produce. The accompanying figures only show the superficial muscles. Some of the muscles discussed in the narrative are deep muscles and thus are not illustrated.

1. Review the muscles involved in each action.
2. Write the names of the muscles in the blanks. The answers are in Appendix I at the back of the book.

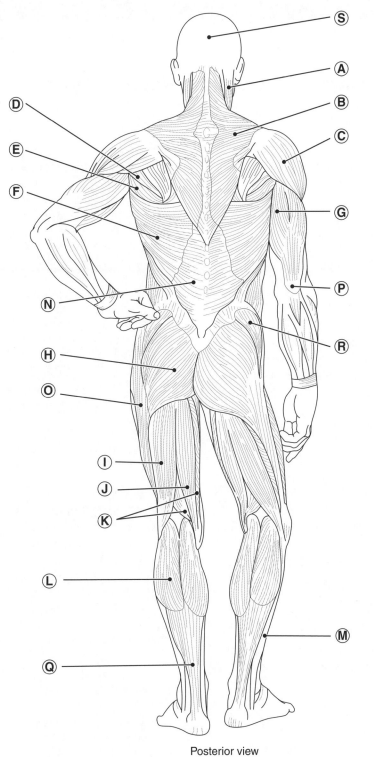

Posterior view

A. _____

B. _____

C. _____

D. _____

E. _____

F. _____

G. _____

H. _____

I. _____

J. _____

K. _____

L. _____

M. _____

N. _____

O. _____

P. _____

Q. _____

R. _____

S. _____

Coloring Exercise 5-1 ➤ Organization of the Nervous System

Anatomical Organization

- **Central nervous system** Ⓐ
  - **Brain** Ⓑ
  - **Spinal cord** Ⓒ
- **Peripheral nervous system** Ⓓ
  - **Spinal nerves** Ⓔ project from the spinal cord
  - **Cranial nerves** Ⓕ project from the brain (see Coloring Exercise 5-10)

Functional Organization

- Autonomic nervous system
  - Controls involuntary functions (heartbeat, stomach movements, enzyme secretion)
  - Divided into sympathetic and parasympathetic divisions (see Coloring Exercise 5-11)
- Somatic nervous system
  - Controls voluntary movements by skeletal muscles (see Coloring Exercise 4-2)

Components

- **Sensory receptors** Ⓖ (skin, eye, nose, ear, tongue; see Chapter 6) collect sensory information
- **Sensory (afferent) neurons** Ⓗ convey information to the brain and spinal cord (CNS)
- CNS (**brain** Ⓑ and **spinal cord** Ⓒ) integrates information and issues commands
- Efferent nerves transmit commands
  - **Autonomic nerves** Ⓘ
  - **Motor nerves** Ⓙ
- Effectors carry out commands
  - **Autonomic effectors** Ⓚ: heart muscle, smooth (visceral) muscle, glands
  - Motor effectors: **skeletal muscles** Ⓛ

COLORING INSTRUCTIONS

Color each structure and its name at the same time, using the same color. On the top figure:

1. Use related, light colors to shade brain Ⓑ and spinal cord Ⓒ.
2. Use related, darker colors to shade the spinal nerves Ⓔ and cranial nerves Ⓕ. Note that the cranial nerves connect with the nose, eyes, or brainstem.

COLORING INSTRUCTIONS

On the bottom figure:

1. Color the letters "CNS" Ⓐ and "PNS" Ⓓ.
2. Color the five examples of sensory receptors Ⓖ and the afferent nerve Ⓗ.
3. Color the brain Ⓑ and spinal cord Ⓒ.
4. Color the autonomic Ⓘ and motor nerves Ⓙ.
5. Color the three examples of autonomic effectors Ⓚ and the skeletal muscle Ⓛ.

Posterior view

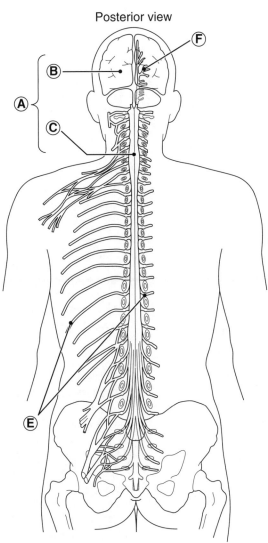

A. central nervous system
B. brain
C. spinal cord
D. peripheral nervous system
E. spinal nerves
F. cranial nerves
G. sensory receptors
H. sensory (afferent) neurons
I. autonomic nerves
J. motor nerves
K. autonomic effectors
L. skeletal muscle

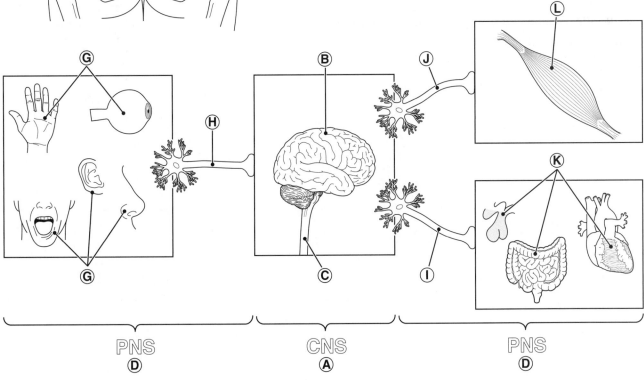

PNS
Ⓓ

CNS
Ⓐ

PNS
Ⓓ

Coloring Exercise 5-2 ➤ Nervous Tissue

Nervous Tissue

- Consists of neurons and neuroglial cells

Neurons: Convey Electrical Signals

- **Cell body** (A)
  - Contains **nucleus** (B), other organelles
  - Receives signals from **dendrites** (C)
  - Sends signals down **axons** (D)
- **Dendrites** (C)
  - Highly branched extensions of the cell body
  - Receive information from receptors (see Coloring Exercise 5-1) and other neurons
  - Conduct nerve impulses **toward** the cell body (C1)
- **Axon** (D)
  - Conducts impulses **away from** cell body (D1), to a **muscle cell** (E), gland, or another neuron
  - May have many branches
  - Sometimes covered in a **myelin sheath** (F) to accelerate transmission (Coloring Exercise 5-4)
    - Myelin synthesized by Schwann cells or oligodendrocytes (see below)
    - Gaps between adjacent myelin sheaths are called **nodes** (G)

Neuroglia: Support and Protect the Neurons

- **Ependymal cells** (H): form cerebrospinal fluid (Coloring Exercise 5-8)
- **Astrocytes** (I): provide nutrients, take up waste products, sometimes produce new neurons
- **Microglia** (J): engulf and degrade microbes and debris
- **Oligodendrocytes** (K): myelinate neurons in the central nervous system
  - Schwann cells myelinate peripheral neurons

COLORING INSTRUCTIONS

Color each structure and its name at the same time, using the same color. On the left figure:

1. Color the parts of the motor neuron and the muscle fiber ((A) to (G)). Draw circles to indicate the nodes (G).
2. Color the arrows representing the transmission of nerve impulses ((C1) and (D1)). Use the same color for (C1) that you used for (C), and the same color for (D1) that you used for (D).

COLORING INSTRUCTIONS

On the right figure:

1. Color the parts of the neuron ((A) to (D), (F)).
2. Color the neuroglia ((H) to (K)), including all four astrocytes (I). Use a similar color for the oligodendrocyte (K) and the myelin sheath (F) to highlight the relationship between these two structures.

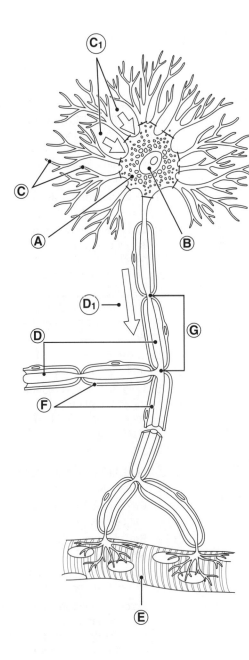

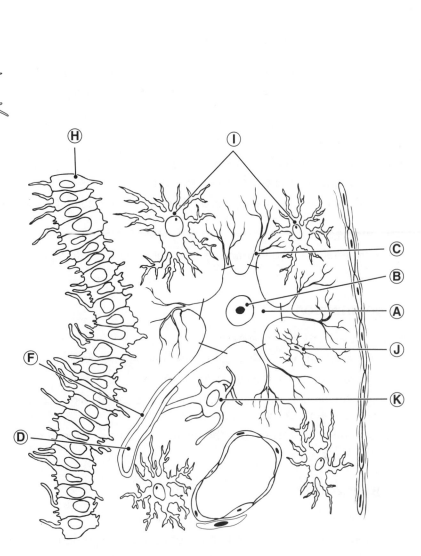

A. cell body
B. nucleus
C. dendrites
C$_1$. towards
D. axon
D$_1$. away from
E. muscle cell
F. myelin sheath
G. node

H. ependymal cell
I. astrocytes
J. microglial cell
K. oligodendrocyte

Coloring Exercise 5-3 ➤ The Action Potential

Resting Membrane Potential Ⓐ

- Membrane potential varies between cells (−60 mV to −70 mV)
- Large **sodium** (**Na+** Ⓑ) and **potassium** (**K+** Ⓒ) gradients
  - Na+ more concentrated outside cell
  - K+ more concentrated inside cell

Electric Gradient

- More **positive ions (+)** Ⓓ outside the cell
- More **negative ions (–)** Ⓔ inside the cell
- Electric gradient created by many different ions, including Na+ and K+

Channels

- **Na channels** Ⓕ and **K channels** Ⓖ involved in the action potential are closed

Depolarization Ⓗ

- Stimulus opens Na+ channels
- Na+ enters cell, increasing number of positive ions inside the cell
- Membrane potential thus becomes positive
- During the action potential, electric gradients change significantly but concentration gradients do not
- Depolarization spreads down the neuron, creating a nerve impulse (Coloring Exercise 5-4)

Repolarization Ⓘ

- Potassium channels open, sodium channels close
- K+ leaves cell, reducing the number of positive ions inside the cell
- Membrane potential becomes negative, returning to rest

Summary

- Concentration gradients do not significantly change during the action potential (they are too large)
- The electric gradient reverses during depolarization
- Sodium channels open to depolarize the membrane, potassium channels open to repolarize the membrane

---

✎ **COLORING INSTRUCTIONS**

Color each part and its name at the same time, using the same color. On the bottom left-hand figure:

1. Color the term "resting membrane potential" Ⓐ.
2. Color the symbols representing Na+ Ⓑ and K+ Ⓒ. The size of the letters reflects the concentration of the ion.
3. Color the symbols indicating the electric gradient (Ⓓ and Ⓔ).
4. Color the closed Na Ⓕ and K Ⓖ channels.
5. Color the line representing the resting membrane potential Ⓐ on top figure.

✎ **COLORING INSTRUCTIONS**

On the middle figure:

1. Color the term "depolarization" Ⓗ.
2. Repeat steps 2 and 3 above.
3. Color the open Na Ⓕ and closed K Ⓖ channels.
4. Color the line representing the membrane potential Ⓗ during depolarization on top figure.

✎ **COLORING INSTRUCTIONS**

On the right-hand figure:

1. Color the term "repolarization" Ⓘ.
2. Repeat steps 2 and 3 above.
3. Color the open Na Ⓕ and closed K Ⓖ channels.
4. Color the line representing the membrane potential during repolarization Ⓘ on the top figure.

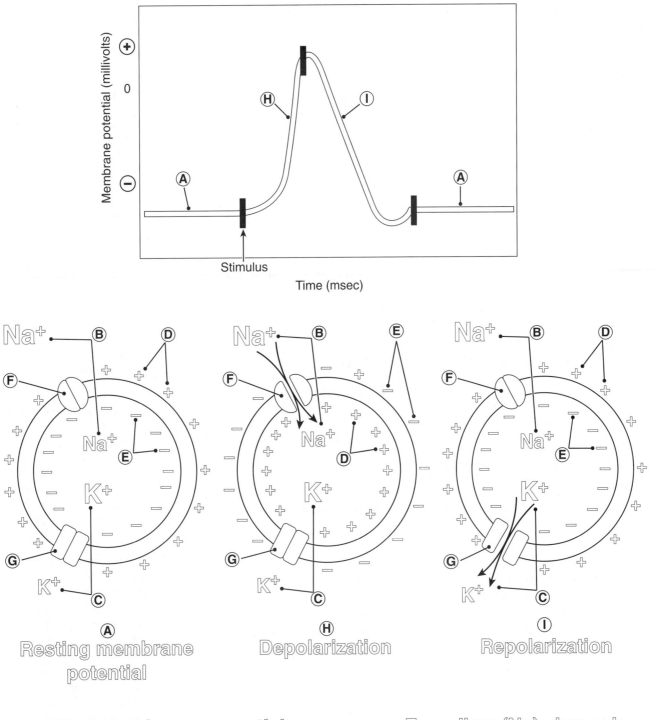

A. resting membrane potential
B. sodium (Na⁺)
C. potassium (K⁺)
D. positive ions (+)
E. negative ions (–)

F. sodium (Na) channels
G. potassium (K) channels
H. deplolarization
I. repolarization

Coloring Exercise 5-4 ➤ Transmission of Nerve Impulses

Transmission Within Neurons

- No action potential: net **positive charge** Ⓐ outside, net **negative charge** Ⓑ inside the neuron
- **Action potential** (Coloring Exercise 5-3) Ⓒ results in DEPOLARIZATION
  - Net positive charge Ⓐ₁ inside neuron, net negative charge Ⓑ outside neuron
- Depolarization triggers action potential in neighboring membrane areas; electrical impulse spreads down the axon (from neuron depiction 1 to depiction 2 to depiction 3)

Myelin

- **Myelin** Ⓓ (Coloring Exercise 5-1) accelerates action potential transmission
  - Myelin prevents action potentials
  - Action potentials jump between nodes, where myelin is absent
  - Fewer action potentials are generated; transmission is faster

Transmission Between Neurons: The Synapse

- Synapse: junction between a neuron and another cell (neuron, muscle...)
  - **Presynaptic cell** Ⓔ: conveys signal
  - **Postsynaptic cell** Ⓕ: receives signal

Chemical Synapses

- **Action potential** Ⓒ depolarizes the **axon end bulb membrane** Ⓔ₁ of the presynaptic cell
- Action potential induces **vesicles** Ⓖ to release **neurotransmitters** Ⓗ into the **synaptic cleft** Ⓘ
- Neurotransmitters bind to **receptors** Ⓙ on postsynaptic cell membrane
- Neurotransmitter-bound receptor causes electric event in postsynaptic cell
  - Depolarization: increases possibility of action potential
  - Hyperpolarization: decreases possibility of action potential
- Postsynaptic cell receives inputs from many presynaptic cells
  - Cell response (action potential or not) determined by sum of ALL inputs
- **Mitochondria** Ⓚ provide energy, synthesize some neurotransmitters

---

COLORING INSTRUCTIONS

Color each part and its name at the same time, using the same color. On the top left figure: color all the elements of one neuron before starting the next neuron.

1. Color the positive Ⓐ and negative Ⓑ charges.
2. Color the positive charges inside the neuron resulting from the action potential Ⓐ₁.
3. Using a light color, color the depolarized portion of the neuron and the arrow representing the action potential Ⓒ.

COLORING INSTRUCTIONS

On the top right figure: color the elements of one neuron before starting the next neuron.

1. Color the myelin sheath Ⓓ.
2. Repeat steps 1–3 above.

COLORING INSTRUCTIONS

Color both parts of bottom figure at the same time.

1. Color the membranes of the presynaptic cell Ⓔ, Ⓔ₁ and the postsynaptic cell Ⓕ.
2. Color the mitochondria Ⓚ wherever you see them.
3. Color the arrow Ⓒ representing the action potential.
4. Use a dark color for the neurotransmitters Ⓗ and a lighter color for the vesicles Ⓖ and synaptic cleft Ⓘ.
5. Color the neurotransmitter receptors Ⓙ.

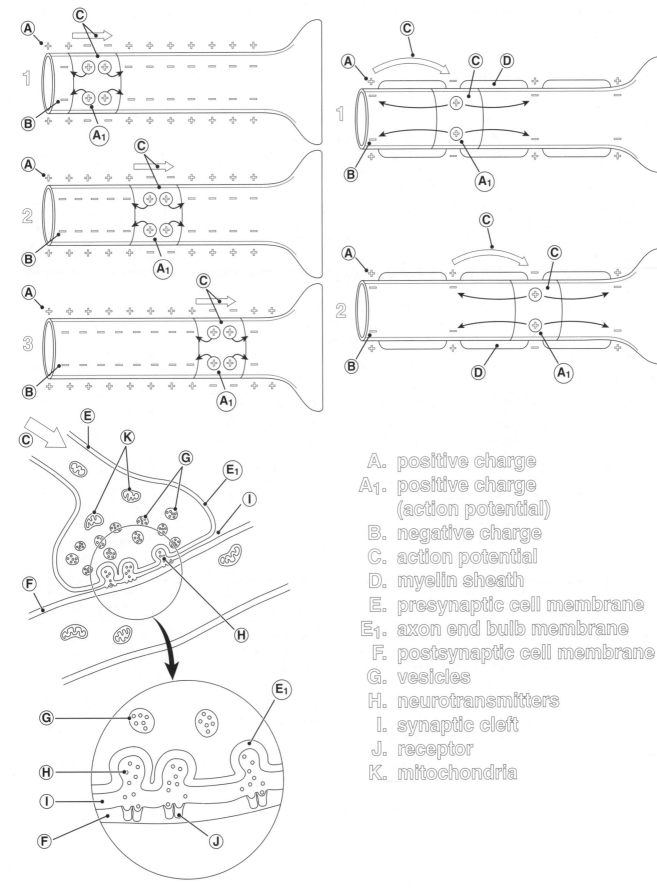

A. positive charge
A_1. positive charge
(action potential)
B. negative charge
C. action potential
D. myelin sheath
E. presynaptic cell membrane
E_1. axon end bulb membrane
F. postsynaptic cell membrane
G. vesicles
H. neurotransmitters
I. synaptic cleft
J. receptor
K. mitochondria

Coloring Exercise 5-5 ➤ The Spinal Cord and Spinal Reflexes

Cross-Section of the Spinal Cord

- **Gray matter** (A) middle: unmyelinated tissue (neuron cell bodies, short unmyelinated axons)
  - Contains right and left sides joined by the **gray commissure** (A1)
  - **Central canal** (B): contains cerebrospinal fluid (see Coloring Exercise 5-8)
  - **Dorsal horns** (A2): entry point for sensory nerves
  - **Ventral horns** (A3): exit point for motor nerves
- **White matter** (C) outside: myelinated axons
  - **Posterior median sulcus** (C1) divides left and right portions posteriorly
  - **Anterior median fissure** (C2) divides left and right portions anteriorly
- **Spinal nerves** (D)
  - Sensory neurons pass through the **dorsal root ganglion** (D1) and the **dorsal root** (D1)
  - Motor neurons pass through the **ventral root** (D3)
  - Ventral and dorsal roots merge to form the spinal nerve (D)
  - Spinal nerve branches into anterior and posterior portions

Spinal Reflexes

Component	Structure	Function	Example
Receptor (E)	Nerve ending, sense organ (e.g., eye)	Detects stimulus	**Pain receptor** (E) detects poking pin
Sensory (afferent) **neuron** (F)	Long dendrite extends from receptor; **cell body** (G) in **dorsal root ganglion** (D1); axon passes through dorsal root into **dorsal horn** (A2)	Conveys stimulus to CNS	**Sensory neuron** (F) conveys response from finger to spinal cord
Integrating Center (H)	Spinal cord interneuron	Integrates information	Single **interneuron** (H) links afferent and efferent neurons
Motor (efferent) **neuron** (I)	Cell body in gray matter; axon leaves **ventral horn** (A3) through the **ventral root** (D3)	Transmits commands from spinal cord	**Motor neuron** (I) travels to biceps brachii muscle
Effector (J)	Muscle or gland (autonomic nervous system only)	Carries out command	**Biceps brachii** (J) contracts; arm moves away from pin

✎ **COLORING INSTRUCTIONS**

Color each part and its name at the same time, using the same color. On the top figure: make sure you color both the left and the right sides.

1. Color the gray commissure (A1), both dorsal horns (A2) and both ventral horns (A3), using one color or closely related colors.

2. Use a dark color for the central canal (B).

3. Color the white matter (C) within the spinal cord; use related, darker colors to outline the posterior median sulcus (C1) and the anterior median fissure (C2).

4. Color the spinal nerves (D), the dorsal root ganglia (D1), and the rest of the dorsal roots (D2) using related colors. Color the ventral roots (D3).

✎ **COLORING INSTRUCTIONS**

On the bottom figure:

1. Lightly shade the parts of the spinal cord and nerve (A2), (A3), (D), (D1), (D2), (D3), using the same colors as above.

2. Use one dark color to shade in the receptor (E), sensory nerve (F), and sensory nerve cell body (G).

3. Color the interneuron (H), the motor neuron (I), and the muscle (J).

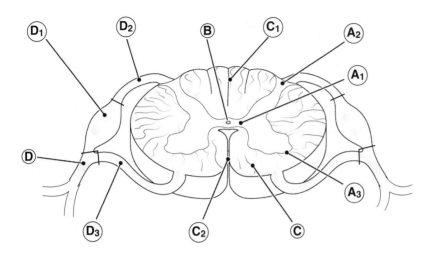

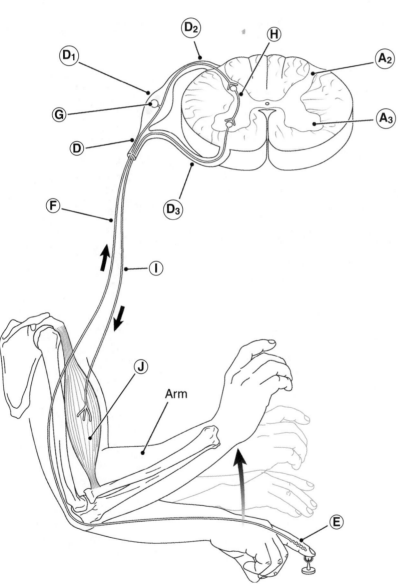

A. gray matter
A₁. gray commissure
A₂. dorsal horn
A₃. ventral horn
B. central canal
C. white matter
C₁. posterior median sulcus
C₂. anterior median fissure
D. spinal nerve
D₁. dorsal root ganglion
D₂. dorsal root
D₃. ventral root
E. receptor
F. afferent/sensory neruon
G. cell body
H. integrating center (interneuron)
I. efferent/motor neuron
J. effector (muscle)

Arm

Coloring Exercise 5-6 ➤ The Spinal Nerves

Spinal Nerves

- Remember that the **brain** Ⓐ, **brainstem** Ⓑ, and **spinal cord** Ⓒ are part of the central nervous system; spinal nerves are part of the peripheral nervous system
- Look back at the top figure on Coloring Exercise 5-5—note that spinal nerves leave either side of the spinal cord and split into anterior and posterior branches
- All spinal nerves are mixed (motor and sensory) nerves
- Nerves are named after vertebrae from which they emerge
  - Eight **cervical nerves** (C1 to C8) Ⓓ
  - Twelve **thoracic nerves** (T1 to T12) Ⓔ
  - Five **lumbar nerves** (L1 to L5) Ⓕ
  - Five **sacral nerves** (S1 to S5) Ⓖ
  - One **coccygeal nerve** (C0) Ⓗ
  - Mnemonic: breakfast at 8 (cervical), lunch at 12 (thoracic), supper at 5 (lumbar, sacral) (from the Memory Notebook of Nursing, Volume II)

Nerve Plexuses

- Anterior branches of most spinal nerves interlace into nerve networks—plexuses
- Thoracic nerves T2 to T11 (**intercostal nerves** Ⓘ) do not form networks
  - Supply the intercostal muscles (Coloring Exercise 4-7)

Plexus	Originating Nerves	Body Regions	Important Branches
Cervical Ⓙ	C1 to C5	Neck, back of head	**Phrenic** Ⓙ1: regulates diaphragm
Brachial Ⓚ	C5 to C7, T1	Upper limb	**Radial** Ⓚ1, **median** Ⓚ2, **ulnar** Ⓚ3
Lumbosacral Ⓛ	T12 to L5, S1 to S5	Pelvis and legs	**Femoral** Ⓛ1, **sciatic** Ⓛ2

✍ **COLORING INSTRUCTIONS**

Color each part and its name at the same time, using the same color.

1. Color the brain Ⓐ, brainstem Ⓑ and/or spinal cord Ⓒ on both figures, using any combination of gray, light brown, and dark brown. Avoid coloring the nerves extending from the spinal cord.

2. On the left-hand figure and on the right side of the spinal column of the right-hand figure, color the nerves using the following color scheme:

   Ⓓ Cervical nerves: yellow

   Ⓔ Thoracic nerves: red

   Ⓕ Lumbar nerves: blue

   Ⓖ Sacral nerves: green

   Ⓗ Coccygeal nerve: purple

✍ **COLORING INSTRUCTIONS**

1. On the left side of the spinal column of the right-hand figure, color the nerve plexuses as follows:

   Cervical plexus Ⓙ: dark yellow

   Brachial plexus Ⓚ: orange

   Intercostal nerves Ⓘ: pink

   Lumbosacral plexus Ⓛ: blue-green

2. Some specific nerves in each plexus are labeled. If you like, you can use darker versions of the color used for the plexus to highlight these nerves.

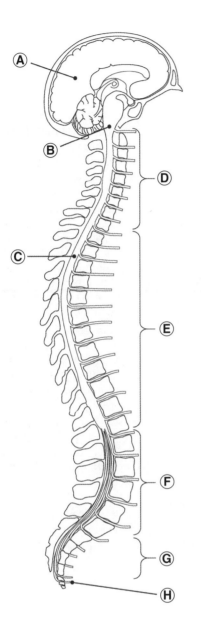

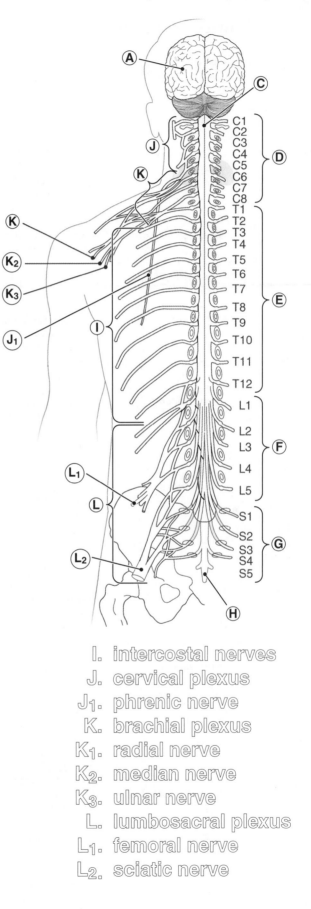

A. brain
B. brainstem
C. spinal cord
D. cervical nerves
E. thoracic nerves
F. lumbar nerves
G. sacral nerves
H. coccygeal nerve

I. intercostal nerves
J. cervical plexus
J₁. phrenic nerve
K. brachial plexus
K₁. radial nerve
K₂. median nerve
K₃. ulnar nerve
L. lumbosacral plexus
L₁. femoral nerve
L₂. sciatic nerve

Coloring Exercise 5-7 ➤ The Brain

Division	Structure	Structure	Function
Cerebrum Ⓐ		Two hemispheres; outer **cortex** Ⓐ1 is gray matter; inner medulla is mostly **white matter** Ⓐ2	Conscious thought, memory, movement, sensation (see Coloring Exercise 5-8)
	Corpus callosum Ⓑ	Axons joining the two hemispheres	
	Basal ganglia (basal nuclei)	Gray matter deep within cerebrum; Includes the **caudate nucleus** Ⓒ, **putamen** Ⓓ, **globus pallidus** Ⓔ	Regulates movement and facial expression; uses the neurotransmitter dopamine
Diencephalon			
	Hypothalamus Ⓕ	Contains many nuclei (collections of neuron cell bodies)	Regulates homeostasis, the **pituitary gland** Ⓖ, reproduction, the autonomic nervous system
	Thalamus Ⓗ	Constitutes most of diencephalon; contains many nuclei	Relays sensory input; involved in movement planning
Cerebellum Ⓘ		Two hemispheres; outer **cortex** (gray matter Ⓘ1), inner **medulla** (white matter Ⓘ2)	Maintains balance and muscle tone
Brainstem			
	Midbrain Ⓙ	Upper portion of brainstem	Controls some reflexes (startle reflex, visual reflexes)
	Pons Ⓚ	Middle portion of brainstem; links cerebellar hemispheres	Breathing control; connects cerebellum with rest of brain
	Medulla oblongata Ⓛ	Continuous with **spinal cord** Ⓜ	Controls vital body functions (e.g., breathing, heartbeat)

✐ COLORING INSTRUCTIONS

Color each part and its name at the same time, using the same color.

1. Color the different brain structures on both figures. Use the same color (perhaps light gray) for Ⓐ and Ⓐ1. Do not color the white matter of the cerebrum Ⓐ2 or the cerebellum Ⓘ2 (leave them white!).

2. Use related colors for the two divisions of the diencephalon (Ⓕ and Ⓗ) and the three divisions of the brain stem (Ⓙ to Ⓛ).

3. Color the pituitary gland Ⓖ using a light color—it is part of the endocrine system (see Coloring Exercise 7-4), not the brain.

4. If you like, lightly shade the rows of the table with the same color used to color the structure.

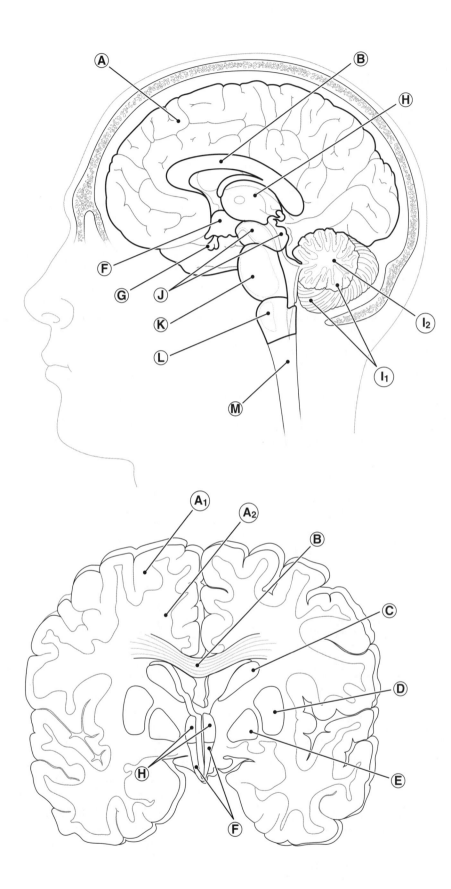

A. cerebrum
A₁. cerebral cortex
A₂. cerebral white matter
B. corpus callosum
C. caudate nucleus
D. putamen
E. globus pallidus
F. hypothalamus
G. pituitary gland
H. thalamus
I. crebellum
I₁. cerebellar cortex
I₂. cerebellar medulla
J. midbrain
K. pons
L. medulla oblongata
M. spinal cord

Coloring Exercise 5-8 ➤ The Cerebral Cortex and the Meninges

Cerebral Cortex

- Surface layer of gray matter
- The cerebrum (including the cortex) is divided into four lobes, based on brain landmarks
  - **Central sulcus** Ⓐ divides frontal, parietal lobes
  - **Lateral sulcus** Ⓑ defines temporal lobe
- Functional areas are associated with specific tasks
  - Receiving areas receive sensory information
  - Association areas integrate information
  - Motor areas initiate movements

Lobe	Functional Area	Function
Frontal Ⓒ		Reasoning, judgment, planning, personality, etc.
	Primary motor area Ⓓ	Controls skeletal muscles
	Written speech area (E1)	Written language
	Motor speech (Broca) area (E2)	Controls speech muscles; only in left hemisphere
Parietal Ⓕ		
	Primary sensory area Ⓖ	Receives sensory information from skin (touch, temperature)
Temporal Ⓗ		Contains olfactory area (deep, not shown)
	Auditory receiving area (I1)	Detects sounds
	Auditory association area (I2)	Interprets sounds
	Speech comprehension **(Wernicke) area** (I3)	Speech recognition, word meanings; left hemisphere
Occipital Ⓙ		Contains visual association area (not shown)
	Visual receiving area Ⓚ	Receives visual input

Protective Structures

Name	Structure	Function
Skin Ⓛ	Many blood vessels; hair	Warm, waterproof
Cranium Ⓜ (Coloring Exercise 3-6)	Bones covered by **periosteum** Ⓝ (membrane)	Protects brain from physical injury
Three Meninges:		
Dura mater Ⓞ	Two layers; outer layer fused to cranium; **dural sinuses** Ⓟ (large veins) run between layers	Cushions and protects brain; venous blood drains into dural sinuses
Arachnoid Ⓠ	Loosely attached to inner dura mater by weblike fibers; **arachnoid villi** (Q1) project into dural sinuses	Cerebrospinal fluid circulates between arachnoid and pia mater (subarachnoid space)
Pia mater Ⓡ	Follows brain and spinal cord contours	Nourishes brain and spinal cord

---

COLORING INSTRUCTIONS

Color each part and its name at the same time, using the same color. On the top figure:

1. Use dark colors to outline the central sulcus Ⓐ and the lateral sulcus Ⓑ.

2. Lightly color the four lobes of the cerebral cortex, which are divided by heavy lines. Use the following color scheme:

   Frontal lobe Ⓒ: light orange

   Parietal lobe Ⓕ: light purple

   Temporal lobe Ⓗ: light blue

   Occipital lobe Ⓙ: light green

3. Color the primary motor area Ⓓ dark red and primary sensory area Ⓖ dark purple. Note that you will be coloring over your shading of the cerebral lobes.

4. Color the three functional areas of the auditory cortex ((I1) to (I3)) dark blue, the two speech areas (E1) and (E2) dark orange, and the visual receiving area Ⓚ dark green.

5. If you like, lightly shade the rows of the table with the same color used to color the structure.

COLORING INSTRUCTIONS

On the bottom figure:

1. Color the structures that protect the brain, from the most superficial (skin Ⓛ) to the deepest (pia mater Ⓡ).

2. If you like, lightly shade the rows of the table with the same color used to color the structure.

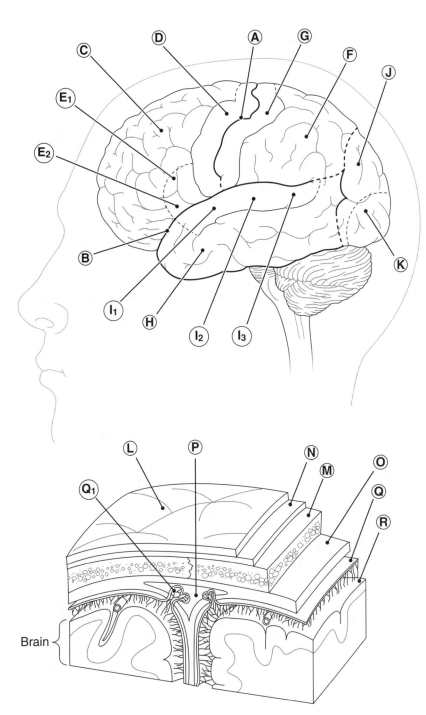

A. central sulcus
B. lateral sulcus
C. frontal lobe
D. primary motor area
E_1. written speech area
E_2. motor speech (Broca) area
F. parietal lobe
G. primary sensory area
H. temporal lobe
I_1. auditory receiving area
I_2. auditory association area
I_3. Wernicke area
J. occipital lobe
K. visual receiving area
L. skin
M. cranium
N. periosteum
O. dura mater
P. dural sinus
Q. arachnoid
Q_1. arachnoid villi
R. pia mater

Coloring Exercise 5-9 ➤ The Ventricles and Cerebrospinal Fluid

Cerebrospinal Fluid (CSF)

- Clear, colorless liquid formed in ventricles
- Cushions brain and spinal cord from mechanical shocks
- Exchanges nutrients, waste products between nervous tissue and blood

Ventricles

- Each lined with **choroid plexus** (Ⓐ, described below)
  - Capillary network
  - CSF formed by filtering blood cells out of blood
- Four ventricles
  - Two **lateral ventricles** Ⓑ
    - One in each cerebral hemisphere
    - **Anterior** Ⓑ1, **posterior** Ⓑ2, and **lateral** Ⓑ3 horns extend into cerebral lobes
  - **Third ventricle** Ⓒ
    - Narrow cavity along the midline of the brain
    - Linked to lateral ventricles by **interventricular foramina** Ⓓ
  - **Fourth ventricle** Ⓔ
    - Linked to third ventricle by the **cerebral aqueduct** Ⓕ
    - Located between the brainstem and the cerebellum
    - Continuous with the **central canal** of the spinal cord Ⓖ (see Coloring Exercise 5-5 and below)

Circulation of Cerebrospinal Fluid

1. CSF forms in the **choroid plexuses** Ⓐ of **lateral ventricles** Ⓑ
2. CSF flows from **lateral ventricles** Ⓑ to **third ventricle** Ⓒ via **interventricular foramina** Ⓓ
3. Third ventricle choroid plexus adds more CSF
4. CSF flows into the **fourth ventricle** Ⓔ via the **cerebral aqueduct** Ⓕ
5. Fourth ventricle choroid plexus Ⓐ adds more CSF
6. CSF flows from the fourth ventricle into the **subarachnoid space** Ⓗ and into the **central canal** Ⓖ of the spinal cord.
7. CSF is reabsorbed via the **arachnoid villi** Ⓘ into large veins; the **superior sagittal sinus** Ⓙ and the **straight sinus** Ⓚ.

✏️ COLORING INSTRUCTIONS

Color each part and its name at the same time, using the same color. On the top figure:

1. Color each structure on both figures. Use the same color for the horns of the lateral ventricles (all of the Ⓑ structures).

2. The interventricular foramina Ⓓ are very small—they join the third ventricle with the lateral ventricles. Use a dark color to highlight the juncture of these ventricles.

✏️ COLORING INSTRUCTIONS

On the bottom figure:

1. Color the choroid plexuses Ⓐ in the lateral ventricle, third ventricle, and fourth ventricle.

2. Work through steps 1–7, coloring structures as you go. Use the same color for the subarachnoid space Ⓗ and the arachnoid villi Ⓘ, and closely related colors for the sinuses (Ⓙ and Ⓚ). The boundaries between structures are not always distinct (for instance, between the third ventricle Ⓒ and the cerebral aqueduct Ⓕ). You can overlap your colors to signify this fact.

3. Trace over the arrows in the subarachnoid space, representing the flow of CSF, using a bright color.

4. Trace over the arrows in the sinuses, representing the flow of blood, using a different bright color.

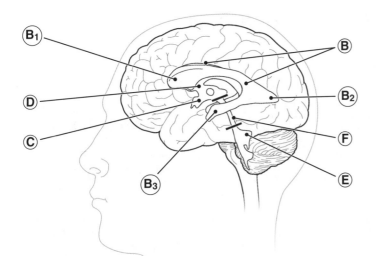

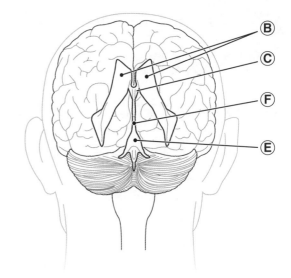

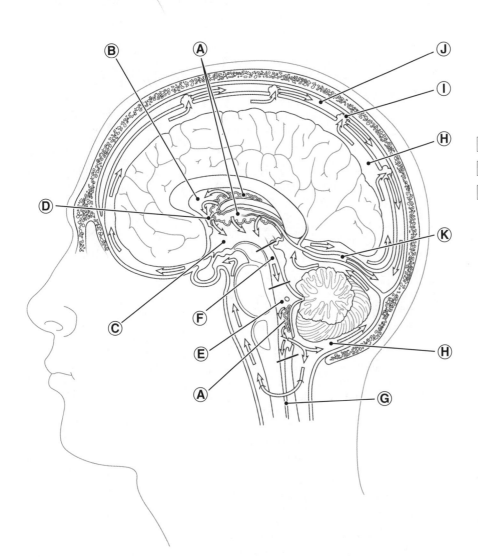

A. choroid plexus
B. lateral ventricles
B₁. anterior horn
B₂. posterior horn
B₃. lateral horn
C. third ventricle
D. interventricular
    foramina
E. fourth ventricle
F. cerebreal
    aqueduct
G. central canal
H. subarachnoid
    space
I. arachnoid villi
J. superior sagittal
   sinus
K. straight sinus

Coloring Exercise 5-10 ➤ The Cranial Nerves

Nerve	Mnemonic*	Name	Sensory Functions	Motor Functions
I Ⓐ	Oh	**Olfactory** Ⓐ	Transmits smell impulses	
II Ⓑ	Oh	**Optic** Ⓑ	Transmits visual impulses	
III Ⓒ	Oh	**Oculomotor** Ⓒ		Controls some external and internal eye muscles
IV Ⓓ	To	**Trochlear** Ⓓ		Controls one eye muscle
V Ⓔ	Touch	**Trigeminal** Ⓔ	Transmits impulses for touch, pressure, pain, and position from the face	Controls chewing muscles
VI Ⓕ	And	**Abducens** Ⓕ		Controls some eye muscles
VII Ⓖ	Feel	**Facial** Ⓖ	Transmits taste impulses from the front of the tongue	Controls muscles of facial expression, some salivary glands
VIII Ⓗ	Very	**Vestibulocochlear** Ⓗ	Transmits impulses for balance and hearing	
IX Ⓘ	Good	**Glossopharyngeal** Ⓘ	Transmits taste impulses and sensations from back of tongue	Controls muscles involved in swallowing
X Ⓙ	Velvet	**Vagus** Ⓙ	Transmits sensations from the throat, thoracic, and abdominal organs	Controls muscles involved in swallowing, coughing, speech; primary parasympathetic nerve
XI Ⓚ	A	**Accessory** Ⓚ	Conveys sensations from the throat	Controls muscles of the larynx, head, shoulders
XII Ⓛ	H!	**Hypoglossal** Ⓛ	Conveys impulses regarding tongue position	Controls tongue movements for swallowing and speech

*Or try: *On One's Own Trying To Acquire Foreign Vocabulary Gives Very Agonizing Headaches.* Daniel Casse, University of Toronto

✐ COLORING INSTRUCTIONS

Color each part and its name at the same time, using the same color.

1. Beginning with Ⓐ, color each cranial nerve and the cartoon(s) indicating movements it controls and/or sensations it transmits. Use related colors for Ⓒ, Ⓓ, and Ⓕ, because they all control eye movements. Color the nerve on both sides of the brain.

2. Using the same color, draw a line between the nerve and the cartoon. Use solid lines for sensory nerves and dashed lines for motor nerves.

3. If you wish, lightly shade the table row with the same color.

A. I olfactory   E. V trigeminal   I. IX glossopharyngeal
B. II optic   F. VI abducens   J. X vagus
C. III oculomotor   G. VII facial   K. XI accessory
D. IV trochlear   H. VIII vestibulocochlear   L. XII hypoglossal

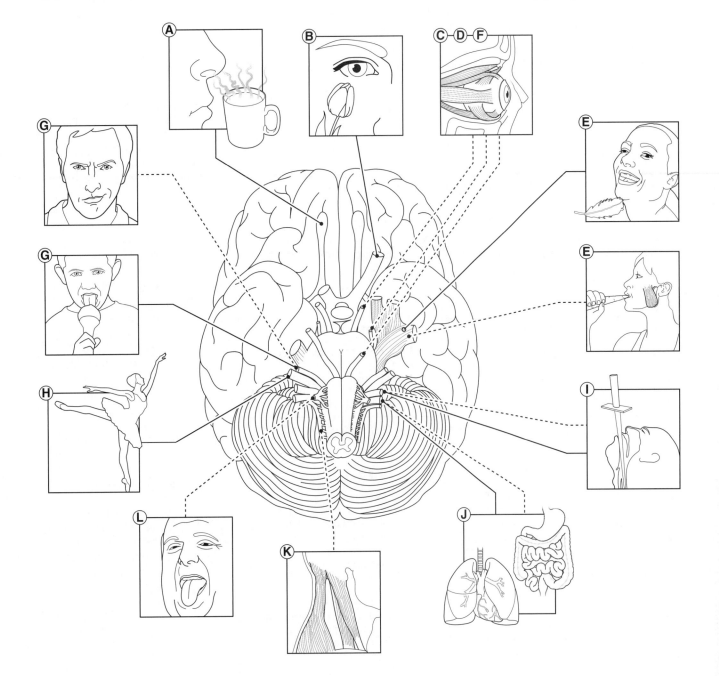

Autonomic Nervous System (ANS)

- Controls involuntary (autonomic) functions
- ANS controls smooth muscles and glands (effectors)
- Each effector controlled by a chain of two neurons
  - Preganglionic fiber: leaves the spinal cord
  - Postganglionic fiber: innervates effector
  - Ganglia: synapses between the two fibers

Divisions

- Sympathetic nervous system: fight-or-flight
  - Spinal nerves T1–T12 and L1–L2
  - Short **preganglionic fibers** Ⓐ, long **postganglionic fibers** Ⓑ
  - Ganglia found near the spinal cord
- Parasympathetic nervous system: rest, digest, and reproduce
  - Cranial nerves II, VII, IX and X, spinal nerves S1 to S3
  - Long (usually) **preganglionic fibers** Ⓒ, short **postganglionic fibers** Ⓓ
  - Ganglia found near the effectors

Effects

Organ	Sympathetic	Parasympathetic
Eye	Dilates pupil	Constricts pupil; produces tears
Salivary glands	Inhibits salivation	Stimulates salivation
Lungs	Dilates bronchi	Constricts bronchi
Heart	Increases heart rate and contraction force	Slows heart rate
Liver	Glucose release	No effect
Spleen	Discharges blood cells	No effect
Stomach and Intestines	Decreases contraction, enzyme production	Increases contraction, enzyme production
Pancreas	Secretes glucagon	Secretes insulin
Kidney	Decreases urine production	None
Bladder	Relaxation	Contraction and emptying
Reproductive organs	Decreases activity (blood vessels constrict)	Increased activity (blood vessels dilate)
Penis	Ejaculation	Erection
Blood vessels (not shown)	Constricts (skin, digestive organs) or dilates (heart, muscles, lungs)	Dilates (digestive organs) or constricts (muscles, lungs)
Skin (not shown)	Perspiration, elevates hairs	No effect

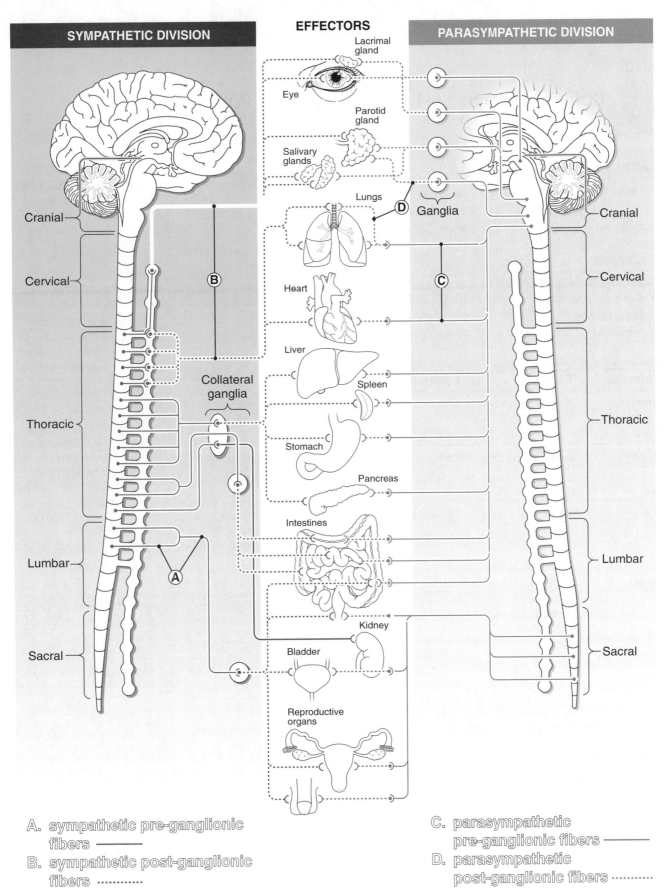

SYMPATHETIC DIVISION

EFFECTORS

PARASYMPATHETIC DIVISION

Cranial

Cervical

Thoracic

Lumbar

Sacral

Collateral ganglia

Lacrimal gland

Eye

Parotid gland

Salivary glands

Lungs

Ganglia

Heart

Liver

Spleen

Stomach

Pancreas

Intestines

Kidney

Bladder

Reproductive organs

Cranial

Cervical

Thoracic

Lumbar

Sacral

A. sympathetic pre-ganglionic fibers ———

B. sympathetic post-ganglionic fibers ··········

C. parasympathetic pre-ganglionic fibers ———

D. parasympathetic post-ganglionic fibers ··········

CHAPTER 6

The Sensory System

Coloring Exercise 6-1 ➤ Touch and Pain

General Senses

- Detect temperature, touch/pressure, pain
- Impulses pass from receptor to the spinal cord (dorsal horn; Coloring Exercise 5-5) and then to the sensory cortex (Coloring Exercise 5-9)

Receptors

- Consist of nerve endings
- Sensory adaptation: receptors that are continually stimulated eventually stop responding
  - Examples: adapting to a hot bath, adapting to the pressure of the seat on your legs

Stimulus	Receptor	Location	Characteristics
Heat (A)	Free nerve ending	Dermis	Detects temperature changes between 90 and 118 F; adapts quickly
Cold (B)	Free nerve ending	Dermis	Detects temperature changes between 50°F and 105°F; adapts quickly
Pain (C)	Free nerve ending	All body tissues	Activated by temperature extremes, mechanical stimuli, chemical stimuli; NEVER adapts
Touch (D)	Tactile (Meissner) corpuscle; nerve endings enclosed by **capsule** (F)	Dermis, around hair follicles	Adapts rapidly
Pressure (E)	Deep pressure receptor (Pacinian corpuscle); nerve endings enclosed by **capsule** (F)	Subcutaneous tissue, near joints and muscles, external genitalia, other sites	Adapts rapidly

Referred Pain

- Pain receptors and visceral organs share common nerve pathways
- Organ pain is perceived in the skin area that shares the pathway
- Some examples are shown in Coloring Exercise 6-1, bottom figure

---

✎ COLORING INSTRUCTIONS

You may want to review skin anatomy (Coloring Exercise 2-1) before coloring this Coloring Exercise. Color each part and its name at the same time, using the same color. On the top figure:

1. Color the receptor, dendrite, cell body, axon, and synapse for the heat receptor (A) all the same color. Use the same color for the photo illustrating the function of the receptor.

2. Repeat step 1 for the other four receptor types ((B) to (E)). Note that cold and heat receptors cannot be distinguished based on appearance.

3. Color the capsules (F) of the touch and pressure receptors.

✎ COLORING INSTRUCTIONS

On the bottom figure, color the sites of referred pain.

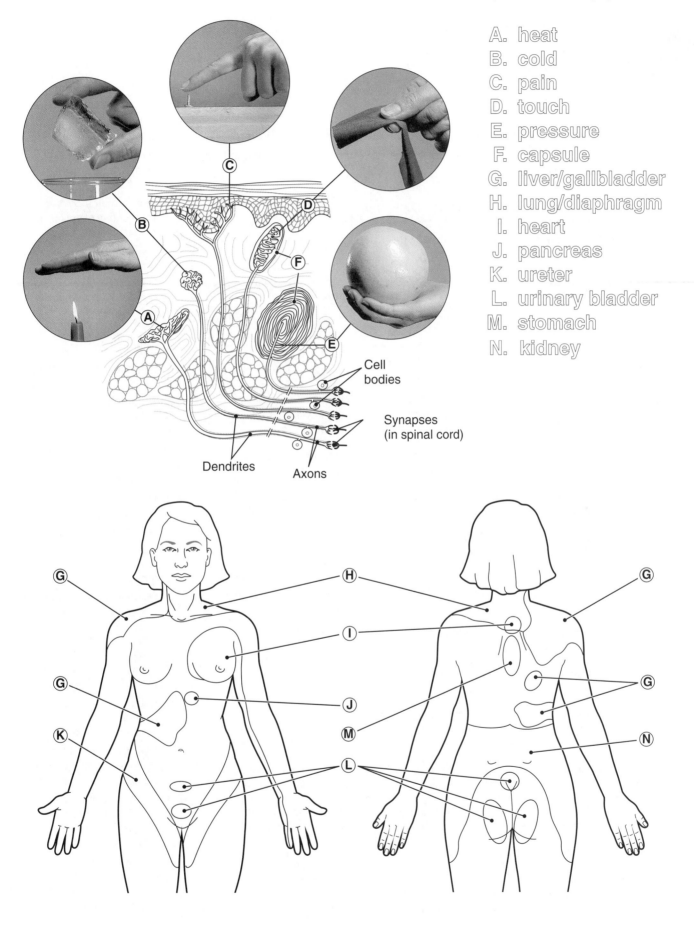

A. heat
B. cold
C. pain
D. touch
E. pressure
F. capsule
G. liver/gallbladder
H. lung/diaphragm
I. heart
J. pancreas
K. ureter
L. urinary bladder
M. stomach
N. kidney

Cell bodies

Synapses (in spinal cord)

Dendrites

Axons

Coloring Exercise 6-2 ➤ The Eye

The Lacrimal Apparatus

- **Lacrimal gland** Ⓐ: produces tears, which flow out through l**acrimal ducts** Ⓐ1
- Tears lubricate the eye, flush away contaminants, and contain substances that defend against microbes
- Tears drain through the:
  - **superior** Ⓑ/**inferior lacrimal canals** Ⓒ into the
  - **lacrimal sac** Ⓓ, which empties into the
  - **nasolacrimal duct** Ⓔ, which opens into the nose

Parts of the Eye

Eye Tunic	Component	Structure	Function
Sclera Ⓕ		Tough connective tissue; no blood vessels; white	Provides support and shape to the eye
	Cornea Ⓖ	Transparent; no blood vessels	The window of the eye; refracts light
Choroid Ⓗ		Delicate connective tissue; many blood vessels; pigmented	Nourishes eye; prevents light rays from bouncing around in the eye
	Iris Ⓘ	Involuntary muscle attached to choroid	Regulates light entry through **pupil** (I1)
	Ciliary muscle Ⓙ	muscle attached to choroid	Controls lens shape (Coloring Exercise 6-3)
	Suspensory ligament Ⓚ	Attaches ciliary muscle to the lens	Controls lens shape (Coloring Exercise 6-3)
Retina Ⓛ		Contains receptors (rods/cones), neurons	Detects light; conveys nerve impulses (Coloring Exercise 6-4)
	Fovea centralis Ⓛ1	Site of many cones	Accurate color vision
	Optic nerve Ⓜ	Nerve connecting retina to brain	Conveys visual impulses to brain
	Optic disk Ⓝ	Where optic nerve, **blood vessels** Ⓞ leave eye	Light rays (and thus images) falling on the optic disk are not detected
Other Structures	**Lens** Ⓟ	Biconvex sphere of elastic material	Refracts light to focus images on the retina
	Aqueous humor Ⓠ	Watery fluid filling the eye anterior to the lens	Maintains the corneal "bulge;" refracts light
	Vitreous body Ⓡ	Jellylike substances filling the eye posterior to the lens	Maintains eyeball shape, refracts light
	Conjunctiva Ⓢ	Lines the inner eyelids and the sclera (not cornea)	Protects eye; produces mucus

---

COLORING INSTRUCTIONS

Color each part and its name at the same time, using the same color. On the left-hand figure:

1. Use the same color for the lacrimal gland Ⓐ and the lacrimal ducts Ⓐ1.
2. Note that the division between the lacrimal sac Ⓓ and the nasolacrimal duct Ⓔ is not distinct. You can overlap your colors to signify this fact.

COLORING INSTRUCTIONS

Read all instructions before you begin coloring. On the right-hand figure:

1. Color each component as you go through the table.
2. Use related colors for the sclera Ⓕ and cornea Ⓖ.
3. Use a dark color for the choroid Ⓗ and the iris Ⓘ. Do not color the pupil (I1).
4. Use contrasting colors for the ciliary muscle Ⓙ and suspensory ligament Ⓚ.
5. Use related colors for the retina Ⓛ and the optic nerve Ⓜ. Use a darker version of the color used for the retina Ⓛ to make a dot at the fovea centralis Ⓛ1.
6. Use a dark color for Ⓝ; outline the circle indicating the optic disk area.
7. Use red to color blood vessels Ⓞ and light colors for structures Ⓟ–Ⓡ.
8. Use a dark color to outline the conjunctiva Ⓢ lining the bottom and upper eyelids.
9. You can color each row of the table with the color used for the structure if you wish.

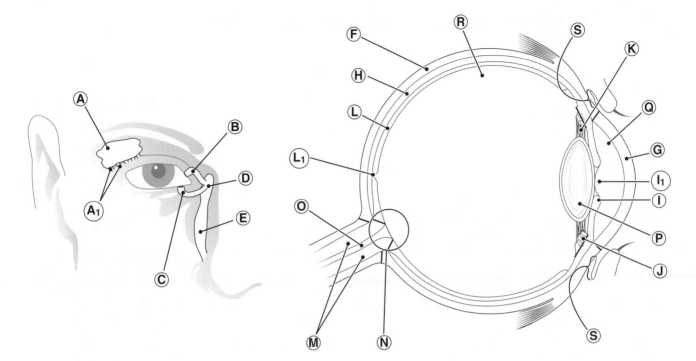

A. lacrimal gland
A₁. lacrimal ducts
B. superior lacrimal canal
C. inferior lacrimal canal
D. lacrimal sac
E. nasolacrimal duct

F. sclera
G. cornea
H. choroid
I. iris
I₁. pupil
J. ciliary muscle
K. suspensory ligament
L. retina
L₁. fovea centralis
M. optic nerve
N. optic disk
O. blood vessels
P. lens
Q. aqueous humor
R. vitreous body
S. conjunctiva

Coloring Exercise 6-3 ➤ Muscles of the Eye

Extrinsic Muscles

- Voluntary muscles attached to outer surface of eyeball
- Eye muscles work together to keep eyes centered on object
- Eye movements
  - **Elevation** Ⓐ1: look up
  - **Depression** Ⓑ1: look down
  - **Abduction** Ⓒ1: look laterally, away from nose
  - **Adduction** Ⓓ1: look medially, toward nose
  - **Lateral rotation and elevation** Ⓔ1: eye rolls up and away from nose
  - **Lateral rotation and depression** Ⓖ1: eye rolls down and away from nose

Name	Origin	Insertion	Action	Nerve
Superior rectus Ⓐ	Tendon ring in eye orbit	Sclera, just superior to the cornea	Elevation	Oculomotor (III)
Inferior rectus Ⓑ	Tendon ring in eye orbit	Sclera, just inferior to the cornea	Depression	Oculomotor (III)
Lateral rectus Ⓒ	Tendon ring in eye orbit	Sclera, just lateral to the cornea	Abduction	Abducens (VI)
Medial rectus (not shown)	Tendon ring in eye orbit	Sclera, just medial to cornea	Adduction	Oculomotor
Superior Oblique Ⓔ	Sphenoid bone in eye orbit	Tendon passes through **trochlea** Ⓕ, inserts in sclera	Lateral rotation and elevation	Trochlear (IV)
Inferior Oblique Ⓖ	Maxilla in eye orbit	Inferior, lateral portion of sclera	Lateral rotation and depression	Oculomotor (III)

Intrinsic Muscles: involuntary

Iris

- Regulates light entry through the **pupil** Ⓗ
- **Circular muscles** Ⓘ: constrict pupil (less light enters)
- **Radial muscles** Ⓙ: dilate pupil (more light enters)

Ciliary Muscles: Accommodation

- Lens refracts (bends) light to focus image on the retina
- More rounded lens = greater refraction

Distance	Ciliary Muscle Ⓚ	Suspensory Ligament Ⓛ	Lens Shape Ⓜ
Near vision	Contracts	Less tension	Rounded*
Far vision	Relaxes	More tension	Flatter

*The lens becomes less flexible with age, and is unable to become round (presbyopia); near vision is impaired.

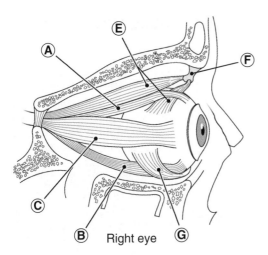

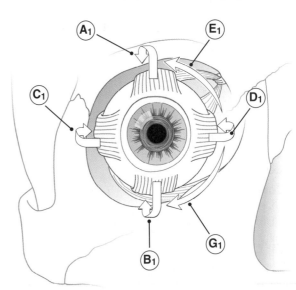

Right eye

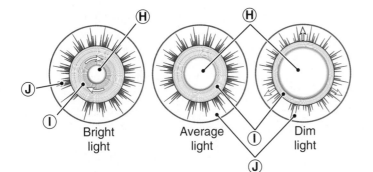

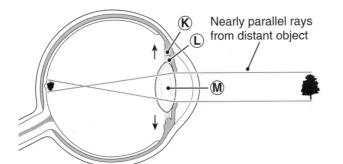

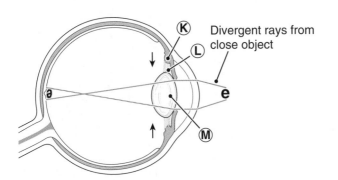

Bright light

Average light

Dim light

Nearly parallel rays from distant object

Divergent rays from close object

A. superior rectus
A₁. elevation
B. inferior rectus
B₁. depression
C. lateral rectus
C₁. abduction
D₁. adduction
E. superior oblique
E₁ lateral rotation/ elevation
F. trochlea
G. inferior oblique
G₁. lateral rotation/ depression
H. pupil
I. circular muscles
J. radial muscles
K. ciliary muscle
L. suspensory ligament
M. lens

Coloring Exercise 6-4 ➤ Vision and Vision Abnormalities

The Retina

- Overlays **choroid** Ⓐ
- **Pigmented layer** of the retina Ⓑ: absorbs stray light waves

Receptor cells

- **Cones** Ⓒ
  - Detect colors
  - Different cones (containing different pigments) detect red, green, or blue light
  - Input from different cones is integrated to detect all possible colors
  - Not very useful in dim light
- **Rods** Ⓓ
  - More sensitive than cones
  - Do not distinguish between different colors
  - Rhodopsin pigment detects light

Physiology of Vision

- **Light rays** Ⓔ pass through retina to activate rods and/or cones
- **Rods** Ⓓ and **cones** Ⓒ activate **bipolar cells** Ⓕ
- Bipolar cells integrate information from neighboring receptor cells (other cells, not shown, also integrate information)
- Bipolar cells activate **ganglion cells** Ⓖ
- Ganglion cell axons form optic nerve (cranial nerve II), convey visual information to visual cortex (see Coloring Exercise 5-9)

Vision Abnormalities: Errors of Refraction

- Remember the **lens** Ⓗ (Coloring Exercise 6-3) bends (refracts) **light rays** Ⓔ to focus images on the retina
- Close vision: light rays bent considerably
- Errors of refraction: light rays are not refracted (bent) correctly, so the **image** Ⓘ of an **object** Ⓙ is out-of-focus

	Myopia Ⓚ **(near-sighted)**	**Hyperopia** Ⓛ **(far-sighted)**
Cause	Eyeball too long	Eyeball too short
Refraction	Excessive	Insufficient
Site of image Ⓘ formation	In front of retina	Behind retina
Close vision	Less impaired	More impaired
Far vision	More impaired	Less impaired
Corrective lenses	**Concave** Ⓜ ("unbends" light rays)	**Convex** Ⓝ (bends light rays more)

✎ **COLORING INSTRUCTIONS**

Color each figure part and its name at the same time, using the same color. On the top figure:

1. Color the parts of the retina and the choroids (Ⓐ–Ⓖ). Do not color the light waves Ⓔ yet.

2. Color the light waves, using a dark color. If you like, color one light wave traveling all of the way through the different layers of the retina.

✎ **COLORING INSTRUCTIONS**

On the bottom figure: Color all of the elements of one image before starting on the next. Begin with the top row. Note that images are projected upside-down on the retina. The brain processes this information, and we perceive the image right side up.

1. Begin with the left hand drawing (uncorrected). Lightly shade the eyeball (Ⓛ). Color the tree Ⓙ and the image of the tree Ⓘ formed near the retina.

2. Color the lens Ⓗ of the eye.

3. Color over the light rays Ⓔ. Use dashed and solid lines.

4. Repeat steps 1 and 2 for the right-hand drawing. Next, color the corrective lens (Ⓝ) before you color the light rays and other elements.

5. Complete all of the steps for the bottom row.

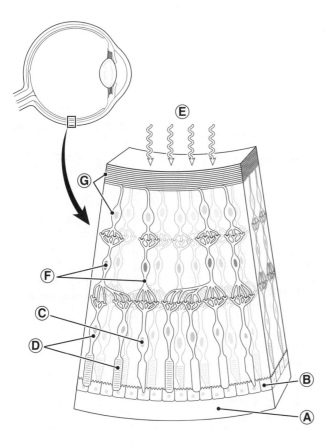

A. choroid
B. pigmented layer
C. cones
D. rods
E. light rays
F. bipolar cells
G. ganglion cells
H. lens
 I. image
 J. object
K. myopia
L. hyperopia
M. concave
N. convex

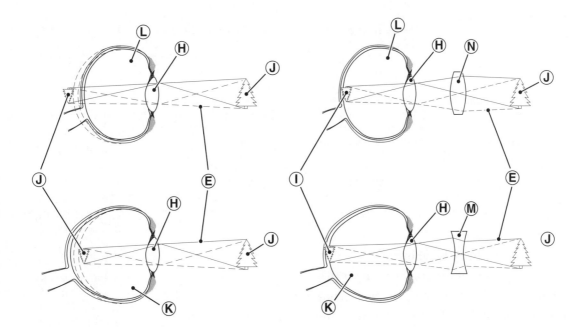

Coloring Exercise 6-5 ➤ Anatomy of the Ear

Anatomy of the Ear

Ear Subdivision	Component	Structure	Function
Outer Ear			
	Pinna Ⓐ	Skin-covered elastic cartilage	Channels sound waves
	External auditory canal Ⓑ	Contains wax-producing glands	Channels sound waves to tympanic membrane
	Tympanic membrane Ⓒ	Thin connective tissue membrane	Vibrates in response to sound waves entering the ear
Middle Ear		Air-filled **cavity** Ⓓ containing ossicles (bones)	**Auditory tube** Ⓔ connects middle ear with **pharynx** Ⓕ
	Malleus Ⓖ	Connects tympanic membrane and incus	Amplifies and transmits sound waves
	Incus Ⓗ	Connects malleus and stapes	Amplifies and transmits sound waves
	Stapes Ⓘ	Connects incus and cochlea	Amplifies and transmits sound waves
Inner Ear		**Vestibulocochlear nerve** Ⓙ (cranial nerve VIIII) transmits impulses to brain	Equilibrium and hearing
	Semicircular canals Ⓚ	Three loops	Equilibrium (Coloring Exercise 6-7)
	Vestibule Ⓛ	Two chambers	Equilibrium (Coloring Exercise 6-7)
	Cochlea Ⓜ	Coiled structure	Hearing (Coloring Exercise 6-6)

The Inner Ear

- Outer bony skeleton (**bony labyrinth** Ⓝ)
- Inner membranous sac (**membranous labyrinth** Ⓞ)
- **Endolymph** Ⓞ circulates in the membranous labyrinth
- **Perilymph** Ⓝ circulates in the space between the membranous labyrinth and the bony labyrinth
- Note that fluids can freely circulate between the semicircular canals, vestibule, and cochlea

COLORING INSTRUCTIONS

Color each figure part and its name at the same time, using the same color. On the top figure:

1. Color the parts of the ear as you read about them in the table.

2. You can color each row of the table with the color used for the component if you wish.

COLORING INSTRUCTIONS

On the bottom figure:

1. Although the semicircular canals Ⓚ, vestibule Ⓛ, and cochlea Ⓜ are labeled, do not color them as you did in the top figure. Instead, color the bony labyrinth, containing perilymph Ⓝ, and the membranous labyrinth, containing endolymph Ⓞ.

2. Color the vestibulocochlear nerve Ⓙ.

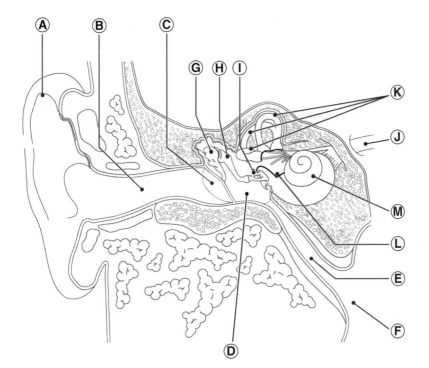

A. pinna

B. external auditory canal

C. tympanic membrane

D. cavity

E. auditory tube

F. pharynx

G. malleus

H. incus

I. stapes

J. vestibulocochlear nerve

K. semicircular canals

L. vestibule

M. cochlea

N. bony labyrinth (perilymph)

O. membranous labyrinth (endolymph)

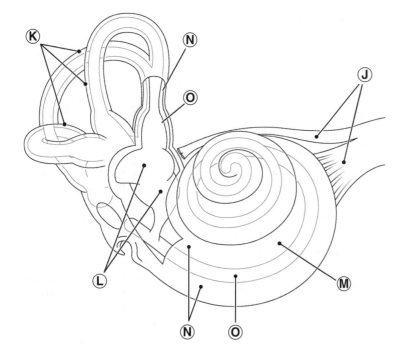

Coloring Exercise 6-6 ➤ Physiology of the Ear: Hearing

The Cochlea and Organ of Corti

- The top figure at right shows a cross-section of the cochlea
- Outer bony labyrinth (containing perilymph)
  - Upper portion: **vestibular duct** Ⓐ
  - Lower portion: **tympanic duct** Ⓑ
- Inner membranous labyrinth (containing endolymph)
  - Called the **cochlear duct** Ⓒ
  - Upper membrane: **vestibular (Reissner) membrane** Ⓓ
  - Lower membrane: **(basilar membrane** Ⓔ**)**
  - Contains the **organ of Corti** Ⓕ
- Organ of Corti contains ciliated **hair cells** Ⓕ₁
  - Hair cells are the RECEPTORS for sound waves
  - Sit on top of the basilar membrane
  - Hair cell cilia embedded in the **tectorial membrane** Ⓖ
  - Send signals to brain via **vestibulocochlear nerve** Ⓗ

Sound Waves

- **High-pitched sounds** (child's voice) Ⓘ: short wavelength
- **Low-pitched sounds** (man's voice) Ⓙ: longer wavelength

Sound Transmission

1. Sound wave vibrates **tympanic membrane** Ⓚ
2. Tympanic membrane vibrates **malleus** Ⓛ, which vibrates **incus** Ⓜ, which vibrates **stapes** Ⓝ
3. Stapes vibrates **oval window** Ⓞ
4. Oval window initiates wave in perilymph of **vestibular duct** Ⓐ
   - Wavelength depends upon the pitch (see above)
5. Wave displaces the vestibular and basilar membranes of the cochlear duct at a characteristic spot
   - **High-pitched sounds** Ⓘ (short wavelength) strike close to the oval window
   - **Low-pitched sounds** Ⓙ (long wavelength) strike far from the oval window
6. Movements of **basilar membrane** Ⓔ bump hair cell cilia against the tectorial membrane (see hair cells and tectorial membrane on the top figure at right)
7. Bumped hair cells send impulses down vestibulocochlear nerve (top figure)
8. Brain interprets the pitch of the sound based on the location of activated hair cells
9. Perilymph wave continues through **tympanic duct** Ⓑ, and is absorbed by vibrations of the **round window** Ⓟ

COLORING INSTRUCTIONS

Color each figure part and its name at the same time, using the same color. On the top right figure:

1. Color the vestibular Ⓐ and tympanic ducts Ⓑ. Use related, light colors, because they both contain perilymph.
2. Color the cochlear duct Ⓒ. Do not color the entire Organ of Corti Ⓕ— just color the hair cells Ⓕ₁.
3. Use dark colors for the vestibular Ⓓ and basilar Ⓔ membranes and to outline the vestibulocochlear nerve Ⓗ.
4. Color the tectorial membrane Ⓖ.

COLORING INSTRUCTIONS

The bottom figure shows a longitudinal view of the cochlea. Compare this figure to the figures in Coloring Exercise 6-5; note that some structures are not shown, and that the cochlea is unrolled. On the bottom figure:

1. Color the tympanic membrane Ⓚ, the three bones of the middle ear (Ⓛ–Ⓝ), and the oval window Ⓞ.
2. Lightly shade the vestibular Ⓐ and tympanic Ⓑ ducts. Note that these two compartments are actually continuous.
3. Color the round window Ⓟ.
4. Color the arrow representing the wave produced by a high-pitched sound Ⓘ.
5. Color the arrow representing the wave produced by a low-pitched sound Ⓙ.
6. Outline the vestibular Ⓓ and basilar Ⓔ membranes, and color the cochlear duct Ⓒ.

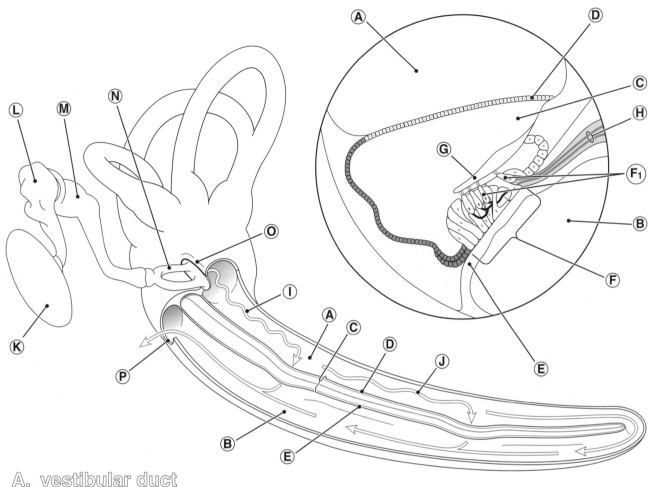

A. vestibular duct
B. tympanic duct
C. cochlear duct
D. vestibular membrane
E. basilar membrane
F. organ of Corti
F₁. hair cells
G. tectorial membrane
H. vestibulocochlear nerve

I. high sound
J. low sound
K. tympanic membrane
L. malleus
M. incus
N. stapes
O. oval window
P. round window

Coloring Exercise 6-7 ➤ Physiology of the Ear: Equilibrium

Equilibrium

- Tells us which way is up, and the direction of head movement
- Two organs of equilibrium
  - **Semicircular canals** (A), containing **cristae** (B)
  - **Vestibules** (C), containing **maculae** (D)
- Organs for equilibrium found within membranous labyrinth, filled with **endolymph** (E) (Coloring Exercise 6-5)
- Note that the membranous labyrinth in the **cochlea** (F) is called the cochlear duct (Coloring Exercise 6-6)
- Signals pass down **vestibular nerve** (G1), which merges with the **cochlear nerve** (G2) to form the **vestibulocochlear nerve** (G3)

Static Equilibrium and Linear Acceleration: Vestibules

Position of head relative to gravity; linear acceleration

Structure of the Vestibules

The membranes of the vestibules (small sacs) contain maculae
- Each macula consists of
  - **Supporting cells** (H)
  - **Receptor cell** (I), with **cilia** (I1)
  - Thick, jellylike fluid (**otolithic membrane** (J)) on top of receptor cells
- **Otoliths** (K) (small stones) rest on top of the thick fluid

Function of the Vestibules

- Head bends forward
- **Endolymph** (E), **otoliths** (K) move under the force of gravity
- **Otolithic membrane** (J) is displaced, bending **receptor cell cilia** (I)
- Receptor cell sends signal down **vestibular nerve fiber** (G)

Rotational Equilibrium: Semicircular Canals

Detects rotation in any plane

Structure of the Canals

- Three canals, perpendicular to each other
- Each canal contains a crista
- Each crista contains
  - **Supporting cells** (H)
  - **Receptor cells** (I), with **cilia** (I1)
- Crista covered by gelatinous **cupula** (L)

Function of the Canals

- Head turns in one direction, creating wave in **endolymph** (E) of one or more semicircular canals
- Endolymph moves **cupula** (L)
- Cupula moves **receptor cell cilia** (I1)
- Receptor cell sends a signal down a **vestibular nerve fiber** (G)

COLORING INSTRUCTIONS

Color each structure and its name at the same time, using the same color. On the view of the inner ear, middle figure:

1. Color the outside of the three semicircular canals (A). Do not color the vestibule (B).
2. Color the endolymph (E) in the membranous labyrinth wherever it is visible—in the semicircular canal, in the vestibule, and in part of the cochlea.
3. Color the crista (B) and the two maculae (D).
4. Color the outside of the cochlea (F).
5. Color all of the nerves (G1)–(G3) the same color.

COLORING INSTRUCTIONS

On the bottom figures, beginning with the left-hand diagram:

1. Color the head, representing static equilibrium (D1) the same color as the maculae (D).
2. Color all of the other structures.
3. Repeat steps one and two for the right hand figure.

COLORING INSTRUCTIONS

On the top figures:

1. Color the ballerina representing rotational equilibrium (B1) the same color as the cristae (B).
2. Color the structures in the left-hand diagram (before rotation).
3. Color all of the structures in the right-hand diagram (after rotation).

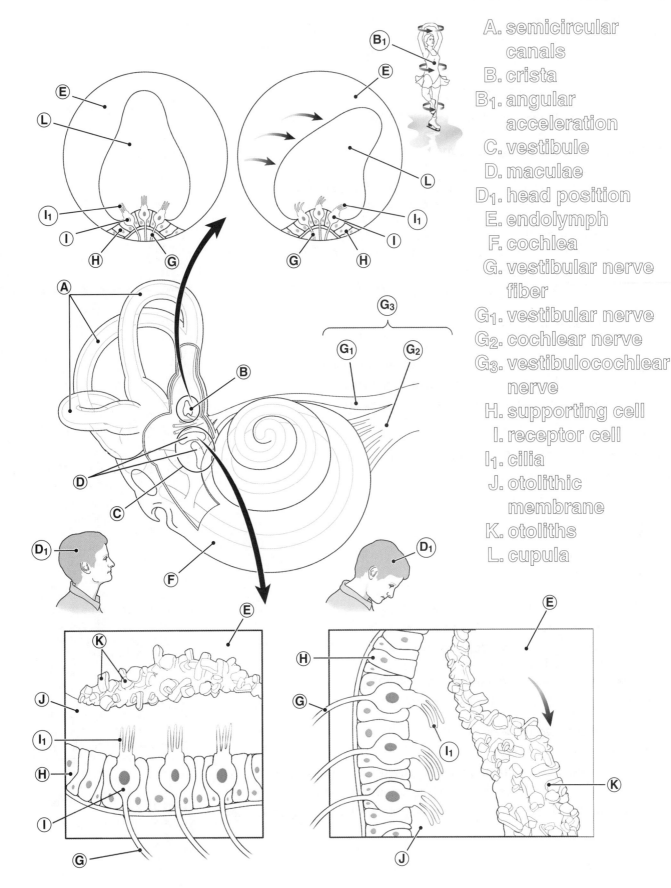

A. semicircular canals
B. crista
B_1. angular acceleration
C. vestibule
D. maculae
D_1. head position
E. endolymph
F. cochlea
G. vestibular nerve fiber
G_1. vestibular nerve
G_2. cochlear nerve
G_3. vestibulocochlear nerve
H. supporting cell
I. receptor cell
I_1. cilia
J. otolithic membrane
K. otoliths
L. cupula

Coloring Exercise 6-8 ➤ The Chemical Senses: Smell and Taste

Smell: The Olfactory Epithelium

Smell "organ," the **olfactory epithelium** (A), is located high up in the nasal cavity

Structure of the Olfactory Epithelium

- **Receptor cells** (B), which are neurons
  - Axon enters brain as part of the **olfactory nerve** (B1) (cranial nerve I); forms synapses with other nerves in the **olfactory bulb** (B2)
  - **Dendrite** (B3) has **cilia** (B4) that bind to odor molecules
  - Humans have about 350 different types of receptor cells, each binding specific odor molecules (and thus detecting different smells)
- **Supporting cells** (C): make mucus
- **Basal cells** (D): produce more receptor cells

Function: The Smelling Process

- Smelly chemical (odorant) dissolves in **mucus layer** (E)
- Dissolved chemical binds to cilia of particular **receptor cell** (B)
- Receptor cell sends action potential up **olfactory nerve** (B1)
- Smell interpreted in the olfactory center of the temporal lobe

Taste: Tongue Taste Buds

- Sensation of taste comes from taste buds, also from smell
- Five basic taste qualities
  - Sweet
  - Salty
  - Sour
  - Bitter
  - Umami (the rich taste found in beef; means "delicious" in Japanese)

Structure

- **Papillae** (F): small or large bumps on the tongue
- The **epithelium** (F1) of each papilla contains **taste buds** (G)
- Each taste bud contains **taste receptor cells** (H)
  - One end projects into **taste pore** (H1)
  - Opposite end synapses with **gustatory neurons** (I)
- **Basal cells** (J) produce new taste receptor cells

Function: The Tasting Process

- Chemical (such as salt) dissolves in saliva
- Dissolved chemical enters **taste pore** (H1), activates **receptor cell** (H)
- Receptor cell induces an action potential in a **gustatory neuron** (I)
- Impulse travels to brain via cranial nerves VII, IX, or X (depending on location of taste bud)

✎ **COLORING INSTRUCTIONS**

Color each structure and its name at the same time, using the same color. On the top figure:

1. On the left-hand diagram, color the olfactory bulb (B2) yellow. Do not color the olfactory epithelium (A); use black to color in the term.

2. On the right-hand diagram, lightly color the mucus layer (E). Color the supporting (C) and basal cells (D).

3. On the right-hand diagram, use yellow (or close variants) for the olfactory nerve (B1), the receptor cell (B), the dendrite (B3), and the cilia (B4).

✎ **COLORING INSTRUCTIONS**

On the bottom figure:

1. Color the papillae (F) on the tongue, noting the different shapes. The largest papillae are found at the back of the tongue.

2. Using the same color, lightly shade the papilla epithelium (F1). Use a dark, contrasting color for the taste buds (G).

3. Color the structures (except the taste pore (H1)) in the magnified view of a taste bud. Use related colors for (G) and (H), since receptor cells make up most of the taste bud.

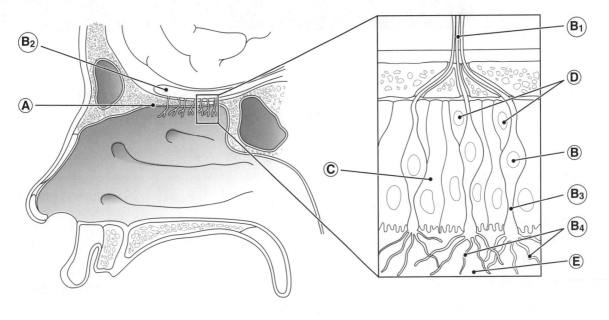

A. olfactory epithelium
B. receptor cell
B_1. olfactory nerve
B_2. olfactory bulb
B_3. dendrite
B_4. cilia
C. supporting cell
D. basal cells

E. mucus layer
F. papillae
F_1. papilla epithelium
G. taste buds
H. taste receptor cell
H_1. taste pore
I. gustatory neuron
J. basal cell

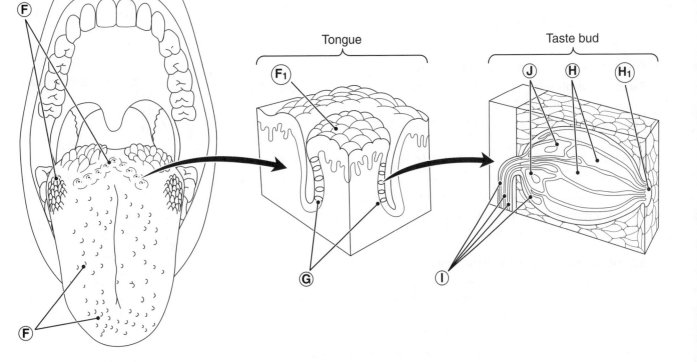

Tongue

Taste bud

CHAPTER 7

The Endocrine System: Glands and Hormones

Coloring Exercise 7-1 ➤ **The Endocrine System and the Endocrine Glands**

The Endocrine System

- Glands containing specialized **endocrine cells** Ⓐ that produce regulatory chemicals (**hormones** Ⓑ)
- Hormones regulate diverse body functions, such as water balance, growth, and reproduction

Hormone Action

- Hormones: chemical messengers that have specific regulatory effects on certain cells or organs
- Mechanism of hormone action:
  - **Endocrine cells** Ⓐ release **hormones** Ⓑ
  - Hormones travel in the **bloodstream** Ⓒ to all body cells
  - Hormones bind specific **receptors** Ⓓ (proteins in the cell membrane, cytoplasm, or nucleus) on **target cells** Ⓔ
  - Hormone-bound receptors affect cell activities (e.g., membrane permeability, metabolic reactions, synthesis of specific proteins, **cell division** Ⓕ)
- Hormones visit every cell, but only affect specific cells
  - **Target cell** Ⓔ possess specific **receptors** Ⓓ that bind the hormone.
  - **Nontarget cells** Ⓖ will have different **receptors** Ⓗ that bind different hormones.

The Endocrine Glands

- Specialize in hormone secretion
- **Thyroid gland** Ⓘ (Coloring Exercise 7-6)
- **Parathyroid glands** Ⓙ (Coloring Exercise 7-2): embedded in the posterior surface of the thyroid gland
- **Adrenal gland** Ⓚ (Coloring Exercises 7-7, 7-8): consists of the **cortex** Ⓚ1 and the **medulla** Ⓚ2
- **Pancreas** Ⓛ (Coloring Exercise 7-3): also regulates digestion (Coloring Exercise 11-5)
- Gonads (**testes** Ⓜ, **ovaries** Ⓝ): primarily involved in reproduction
- **Pituitary gland** Ⓞ (Coloring Exercises 7-4 and 7-5): controls the thyroid gland, adrenal gland, and gonads

Other Hormone-Producing Structures

- **Hypothalamus** Ⓟ, is part of the brain (Coloring Exercise 5-9)
  - Regulates many bodily functions using both the nervous system and the endocrine system
  - Works closely with the pituitary gland
- Other brain parts, thymus, heart, stomach, duodenum, liver, kidney, and skin also secrete important hormones

✎🗋 **COLORING INSTRUCTIONS**

Color each structure and its corresponding term at the same time, using the same color. On the top figure:

1. Color the endocrine cell Ⓐ in a light color, and the blood vessel Ⓒ light red.
2. Color the hormone molecules Ⓑ a dark color in the cell and as they journey in the blood to other cells.
3. Color the target cell Ⓔ and the receptor Ⓓ that binds the hormone.
4. Color the two new cells Ⓕ produced when the hormone binds the receptor.
5. Color the nontarget cell Ⓖ that has receptors Ⓗ that bind a different hormone.

✎🗋 **COLORING INSTRUCTIONS**

Read all instructions before proceeding. On the bottom figure:

1. Color the endocrine glands and other hormone-secreting structures (Ⓘ to Ⓟ).
2. Note that the parathyroid glands Ⓙ are only visible on the pull-out of the thyroid gland (a posterior view).
3. Use related colors for the adrenal gland Ⓚ and its parts Ⓚ1 and Ⓚ2.
4. The pituitary gland Ⓞ and the hypothalamus Ⓟ are very small; use bright, contrasting colors for these structures.

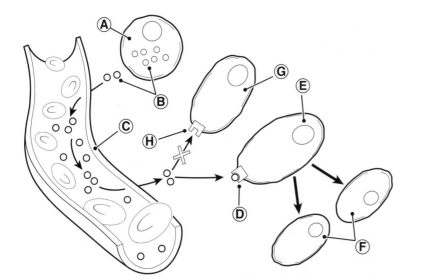

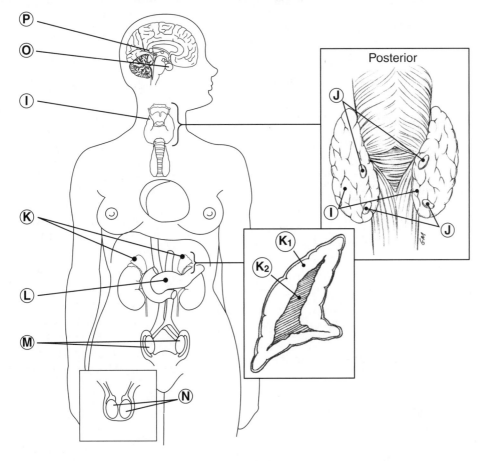

A. endocrine cell
B. hormone
C. blood
D. receptor A
E. target cell
F. cell division
G. non-target cell
H. receptor B
 I. thryoid gland
 J. parathyroid
   glands
 K. adrenal gland
K₁. cortex
K₂. medulla
 L. pancreas
M. ovaries
N. testes
O. pituitary gland
P. hypothalamus

Coloring Exercise 7-2 ➤ The Parathyroid Glands and Calcium Metabolism

Calcium Metabolism

- Blood calcium (**Ca^{2+}** Ⓐ) concentration critical for health
- Ca^{2+} levels determined by events in:
  - **Bone** Ⓑ: bone synthesis reduces ↓ blood Ca^{2+}, bone breakdown increases (↑) blood Ca^{2+}
  - **Kidney** Ⓒ: increased Ca^{2+} retention increases blood Ca^{2+}, increased Ca^{2+} loss (in the **urine** Ⓒ1) decreases blood Ca^{2+}
  - **Intestine** Ⓓ: increased absorption of dietary Ca^{2+} increases blood Ca^{2+}
- Blood Ca^{2+} levels regulated by coordinated actions of three hormones

	Parathyroid hormone (PTH) Ⓔ	Calcitonin Ⓕ	Vitamin D3 Ⓖ
Site of Production	**Parathyroid glands** Ⓗ	**Thyroid gland** Ⓘ	Produced in skin; activated in liver and kidney
Stimulus for Secretion	Low blood calcium	High blood calcium	Parathyroid hormone
Overall Action	↑ Blood calcium	↓ Blood calcium	↑ Blood calcium
Bone Effects	↑ **Bone breakdown** Ⓔ1	↑ **Bone synthesis** Ⓕ1	
Kidney Effects	↑ **Ca^{2+} retention** Ⓔ2	↑ **Ca^{2+} loss** in urine Ⓕ2	
Intestine Effects			↑ **Ca^{2+} absorption** Ⓖ1

Regulation of PTH and Calcitonin Synthesis

- The bottom figure at right illustrates the regulation of PTH and calcitonin synthesis by **negative feedback** Ⓙ
  - Hormone induces a change, and the change inhibits production of the hormone
- The normal blood Ca^{2+} concentration is six diamonds (representing 9–11 mg/100 mL blood)
- Regulation of PTH secretion
  - Low blood Ca^{2+} (four diamonds) stimulates PTH production
  - PTH increases blood Ca^{2+} to normal (six diamonds)
  - PTH secretion is no longer stimulated
  - Note: High blood Ca^{2+} inhibits PTH secretion
- Regulation of calcitonin secretion
  - High blood Ca^{2+} (eight diamonds) stimulates calcitonin production
  - Calcitonin decreases blood Ca^{2+} to normal (six diamonds)
  - Calcitonin secretion is no longer stimulated
  - Note: Low blood Ca^{2+} inhibits calcitonin secretion

✐ **COLORING INSTRUCTIONS**

Color each figure part and its term at the same time, using the same color. On the top figure:

1. Color the calcium ions Ⓐ in the blood. If you wish, color the background of the blood vessel red.
2. Color the organs involved in calcium metabolism (bone Ⓑ, kidney Ⓒ, and intestine Ⓓ). Color both the kidney and the urine Ⓒ1 yellow.
3. Color the hormone names in the terms list (Ⓔ, Ⓕ, Ⓖ), using contrasting colors.
4. Color the arrows, representing the actions of the different hormones. First, color arrows Ⓔ1 and Ⓔ2 using the same color used to color PTH Ⓔ in the terms list. Repeat this process for Ⓕ1, Ⓕ2, and Ⓖ1.

✐ **COLORING INSTRUCTIONS**

On the bottom figure:

1. Color the 4 parathyroid glands Ⓗ. Color the thyroid gland Ⓘ. The sites of vitamin D3 synthesis are not shown.
2. Begin with the left-hand feedback loop, involving PTH.
3. Starting at the top, color the Ca^{2+} ions Ⓐ, and then the hormone name Ⓔ.
4. Color the changed number of Ca^{2+} ions Ⓐ resulting from the hormone action. Finally, color the icon representing negative feedback Ⓙ.
5. Repeat steps 3 and 4 for the right-hand feedback loop, involving calcitonin Ⓕ.

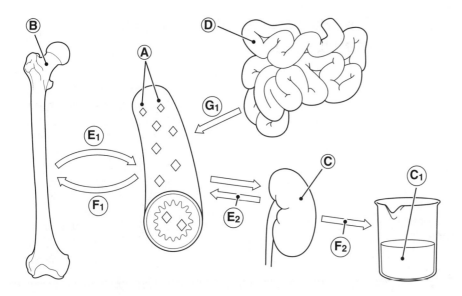

A. calcium (Ca^{2+})
B. bone
C. kidney
C_1. urine
D. intestine
E. parathyroid
   hormone (PTH)
E_1. bone breakdown
E_2. Ca^{2+} retention
F. calcitonin
F_1. bone synthesis
F_2. Ca^{2+} loss
G. vitamin D_3
G_1. Ca^{2+} absorption
H. parathyroid
   glands
I. thyroid gland
J. negative
   feedback

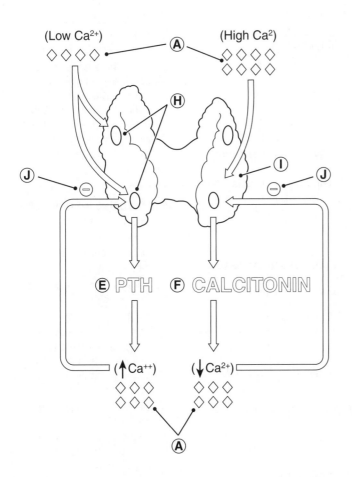

Coloring Exercise 7-3 ➤ The Pancreas and Glucose Metabolism

Glucose

Glucose Ⓐ

- Critical energy source, acquired from
  - Diet (sugars, starches)
  - **Amino acids** Ⓑ (from **proteins** Ⓒ)
  - Fatty acids (from **fats** Ⓓ)
- Blood glucose concentration is tightly regulated
  - Hypoglycemia: insufficient blood glucose
  - Hyperglycemia: excess blood glucose
- Regulated by pancreatic hormones
  - **Insulin** Ⓔ lowers blood glucose levels
    - Cells take up and use glucose to meet energy needs, and store the excess
  - **Glucagon** Ⓕ raises blood glucose levels
    - Liver generates glucose
- Growth hormone, epinephrine, and cortisol also raise blood glucose levels

	Insulin Ⓔ	**Glucagon** Ⓕ
General Effects (**muscle cells** Ⓖ, other cells)	↑ **Glucose uptake** Ⓔ1 ↑ **Glucose breakdown** for energy (ATP) Ⓔ2 ↑ **Synthesis of protein** from amino acids Ⓔ3	
Liver Ⓗ Effects	↑ **Glucose storage** (as **glycogen** Ⓘ) Ⓔ4	↑ **Glycogen breakdown** into glucose Ⓕ1 ↑ **Glucose synthesis** from amino acids Ⓕ2
Adipose Ⓙ Effects	↑ **Fat synthesis** Ⓔ5 from glucose (multistep pathway)	
Site of Production	**Beta cells (pancreas)** Ⓚ	**Alpha cells (pancreas)** Ⓛ
Stimulus for Secretion	High blood sugar (feasting)	Low blood sugar (fasting)
Overall Action	↓ Blood sugar	↑ Blood sugar

Regulation of Insulin and Glucagon Synthesis

- The bottom figure at right illustrates the regulation of insulin and glucagon synthesis by **negative feedback** Ⓜ
- Normal blood glucose concentration: six hexagons (representing 90 mg/100 mL blood)
- Regulation of insulin secretion
  - Hyperglycemia (8 hexagons) stimulates production
  - Insulin decreases blood glucose levels to normal (six hexagons)
  - Insulin secretion is no longer stimulated
- Regulation of glucagon secretion
  - Hypoglycemia (4 hexagons) stimulates production
  - Glucagon decreases blood glucose to normal (six hexagons)
  - Glucagon secretion is no longer stimulated

✐ **COLORING INSTRUCTIONS**

Color each figure part and its name at the same time, using the same color. On the top figure:

1. Color the glucose ions Ⓐ in the blood. Lightly color the organs involved in glucose metabolism (Ⓗ, Ⓖ, and Ⓙ).
2. Color the nutrients wherever they are found; glucose (hexagons Ⓐ), glycogen (hexagon strings Ⓘ), amino acids (triangles Ⓑ), proteins (triangle strings Ⓒ), and fats (ovals Ⓓ). Use related colors for Ⓐ and Ⓘ, and for Ⓑ and Ⓒ.
3. Color the arrows representing insulin actions (Ⓔ1 to Ⓔ5) using the color used for insulin Ⓔ. Color the arrows representing glucagon actions (Ⓕ1, Ⓕ2) using the color used for glucagon Ⓕ.

✐ **COLORING INSTRUCTIONS**

On the bottom figure:

1. Color the beta Ⓚ and alpha Ⓛ cells of the pancreas.
2. Begin with the left-hand feedback loop, involving insulin.
3. Starting at the top, color the glucose molecules Ⓐ. Color the cartoon representing feasting and then the hormone name Ⓔ.
4. Color the changed number of glucose molecules Ⓐ resulting from the hormone action. Finally, color the arrow representing negative feedback Ⓜ.
5. Repeat step 2 for the right-hand feedback loop, involving glucagon and fasting Ⓕ.

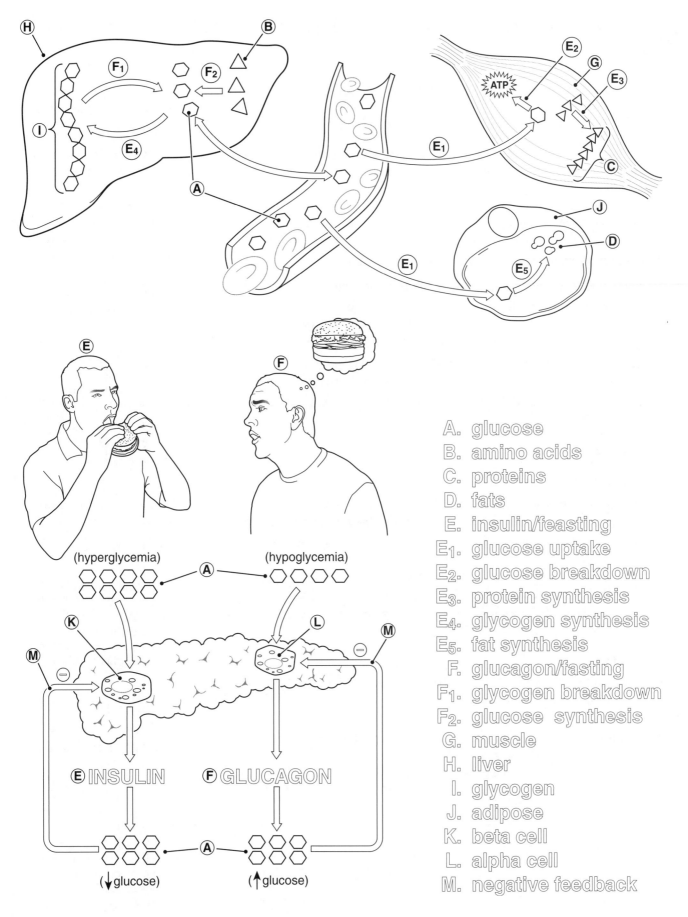

A. glucose
B. amino acids
C. proteins
D. fats
E. insulin/feasting
E_1. glucose uptake
E_2. glucose breakdown
E_3. protein synthesis
E_4. glycogen synthesis
E_5. fat synthesis
F. glucagon/fasting
F_1. glycogen breakdown
F_2. glucose synthesis
G. muscle
H. liver
I. glycogen
J. adipose
K. beta cell
L. alpha cell
M. negative feedback

Coloring Exercise 7-4 ➤ The Pituitary Gland: Posterior Lobe

Structure of the Pituitary Gland (Hypophysis)

- Cherry-sized gland located in a depression of the sphenoid bone, posterior to optic chiasm
- Surrounded by bone, except where it connects with the **hypothalamus** Ⓐ of the brain by the **infundibulum** Ⓑ
- Divided into two parts:
  - **Posterior lobe** Ⓒ: nervous tissue
  - **Anterior lobe** Ⓓ: glandular tissue

The Hypothalamus and the Posterior Lobe

- Posterior lobe is physical extension of the hypothalamus
- Individual **neurons** Ⓔ synthesize and secrete hormones
- Hormones synthesized in the neuron cell body (in the hypothalamus) and secreted from the axon terminal (in the posterior lobe) into **capillaries** Ⓕ
- Capillaries receive blood from an **artery** Ⓖ and drain into a **vein** Ⓗ
- Posterior lobe hormones travel in the blood stream to any site in the body
- Two main hormones synthesized in hypothalamus and released from posterior pituitary gland:
  - **Oxytocin** Ⓘ
  - **Antidiuretic hormone** Ⓙ

Antidiuretic Hormone (ADH)

- Causes water retention
- Promotes the reabsorption of water from the **kidney** Ⓚ into the blood
- Results in reduced volumes of concentrated **urine** Ⓛ, increased volumes of dilute blood
- Released when an individual is **dehydrated** Ⓜ or has low blood pressure (for instance, from bleeding)
- ADH deficiency (**diabetes insipidus** Ⓛ1) causes excessive water loss (large urine volume is produced)

Oxytocin

- Causes contractions of the **uterus** Ⓝ and triggers milk ejection from the **breasts** Ⓞ.
- Used medically to induce labor.
- Secretion stimulated by the pressure of the baby's head on the cervix during childbirth and when a **baby** Ⓟ nurses

---

COLORING INSTRUCTIONS

Color each part and its name at the same time, using the same color.

1. Use light colors to color structures Ⓐ to Ⓓ.
2. Save red, purple, and blue for later.

COLORING INSTRUCTIONS

1. Lightly shade the neurons Ⓔ.
2. Color the hormones (Ⓘ and Ⓙ) as they pass down the neurons. Use orange or brown for Ⓙ.
3. Color blood vessels Ⓕ, Ⓖ, and Ⓗ purple, red, and blue (respectively).

COLORING INSTRUCTIONS

1. Color ADH molecules Ⓙ as they leave the posterior lobe, the kidney Ⓚ, the concentrated urine (Ⓛ, use dark yellow), and the arrow representing the reduced urine volume.
2. Color the cartoon of a situation when ADH secretion will be increased Ⓜ.
3. Color the increased urine volume in a patient with diabetes insipidus Ⓛ1.
4. Use related colors for all of these parts.

COLORING INSTRUCTIONS

1. Color oxytocin molecules Ⓘ leaving the posterior lobe. Color the oxytocin target organs: breast Ⓞ and uterus Ⓝ.
2. Color the cartoon of a situation when oxytocin secretion will be increased Ⓟ.
3. Use related colors for all of these parts.

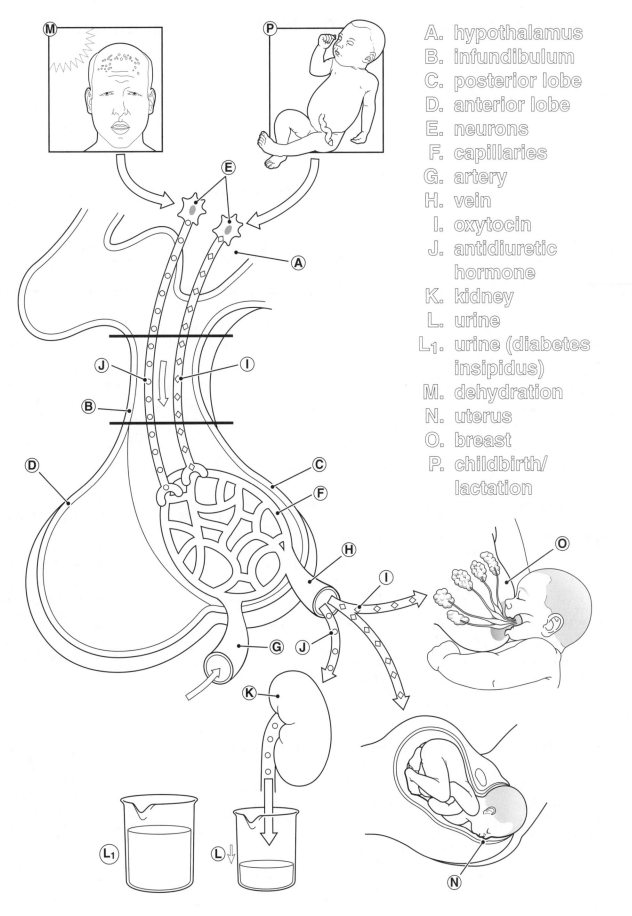

A. hypothalamus
B. infundibulum
C. posterior lobe
D. anterior lobe
E. neurons
F. capillaries
G. artery
H. vein
I. oxytocin
J. antidiuretic
   hormone
K. kidney
L. urine
L_1. urine (diabetes
   insipidus)
M. dehydration
N. uterus
O. breast
P. childbirth/
   lactation

Coloring Exercise 7-5 ➤ The Pituitary Gland: Anterior Lobe

Anterior Lobe and the Hypothalamus

- Remember that the **hypothalamus** Ⓐ is connected to the pituitary gland by the **infundibulum** Ⓑ
- Infundibulum contains neurons extending into the **posterior lobe** Ⓒ and blood vessels extending into **anterior lobe** Ⓓ
- Certain hypothalamic **neurons** Ⓔ control anterior pituitary by **releasing hormones** Ⓕ

Hypothalamic Releasing Hormones

- Released from terminal of short axons into blood vessels (the **portal circulation** Ⓖ)
- Each releasing hormone regulates the production of specific pituitary hormones
  - Releasing hormone named after a hormone they affect (see table, below)
  - Secretion of releasing hormones controlled by negative feedback and neural stimuli (see Coloring Exercises 7-6 and 7-8 for examples)

Hormones of the Anterior Lobe

- Five types of endocrine cells, specializing in the production of a particular hormone, secrete into a **capillary bed** Ⓗ
- Capillaries receive blood from an **artery** Ⓘ and drain into a **vein** Ⓙ.
- Some anterior pituitary hormones act on their target organs to stimulate the production of other hormones.

Hormone	Actions	Releasing Hormones
Growth hormone (GH) Ⓚ	Stimulates growth of **bones, soft tissues** Ⓛ Promotes protein synthesis Increases blood sugar levels Promotes tissue repair	↑: GH releasing hormone (GHRH) ↓: Somatostatin (SRIF)
Prolactin Ⓜ	Stimulates milk production in the **breast** Ⓝ	↓: Dopamine
Thyroid-stimulating hormone (TSH) Ⓞ	Stimulates thyroid hormone production by the **thyroid gland** Ⓟ (see Coloring Exercise 7-6)	↑: Thyrotropin releasing hormone (TRH)
Adrenocorticotropic hormone (ACTH) Ⓠ	Stimulates production of steroids from **adrenal gland** Ⓡ, especially cortisol (see Coloring Exercise 7-8)	↑: Corticotropin releasing hormone (CRH)
Follicle-stimulating hormone (FSH)/ Luteinizing hormone (LH) Ⓢ	Regulates gamete (sperm and egg) production and sex steroid (testosterone, estrogen, progesterone) production from **gonads** Ⓣ	↑: Gonadotropin releasing hormone (GnRH)

A. hypothalamus
B. infundibulum
C. posterior lobe
D. anterior lobe
E. neurons
F. releasing hormones
G. portal circulation
H. capillary bed
 I. artery
J. vein
K. growth hormone
L. bones, soft tissue
M. prolactin
N. breast
O. thyroid stimulating
   hormone
P. thyroid gland
Q. adrenocorticotropin
R. adrenal gland
S. follicle stimulating
   hormone/luteinizing
   hormone
T. gonads

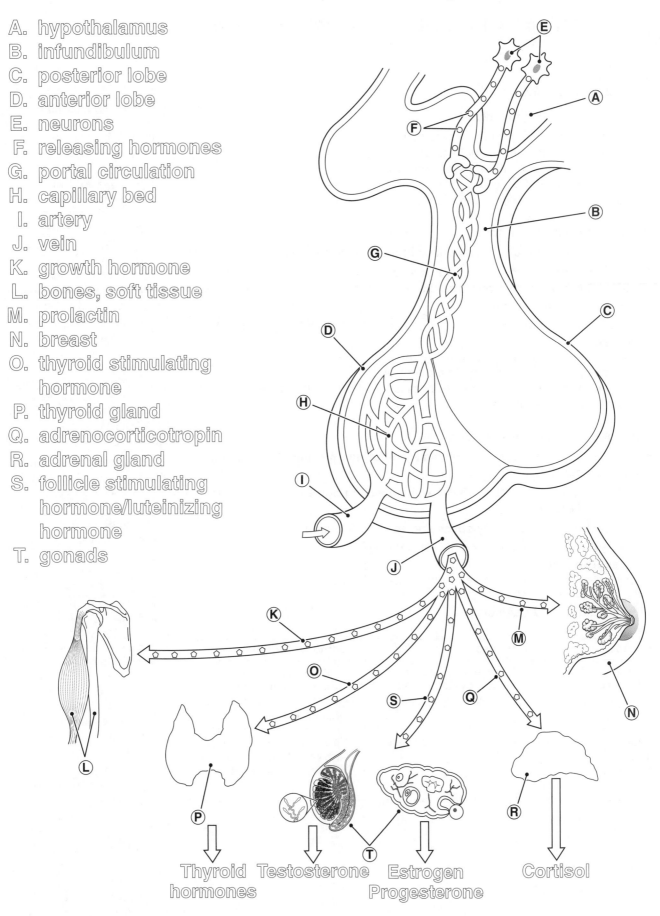

Thyroid   Testosterone   Estrogen   Cortisol
hormones   Progesterone

Coloring Exercise 7-6 ➤ Thyroid Hormones

Thyroid Hormones

- Produced by the **thyroid gland** Ⓑ
- Modified amino acids; contain iodine molecules
  - Thyroxine (T_4, four iodine molecules)
  - Tri-iodothyronine (T_3, three iodine molecules)
  - T_3 is more powerful than T_4, but they exert the same actions
  - T_4 can be converted into T_3 in tissues

Actions of Thyroid Hormones

- Stimulates **growth** Ⓒ and **brain development** Ⓓ in children
- Enhances some effects of the sympathetic nervous system
  - Increases **heart rate**, blood pressure Ⓔ
  - Stimulates **brain activity** Ⓕ
- Increases **metabolic rate** (rate at which cells burn **nutrients** Ⓖ to produce **energy** Ⓗ)
  - More energy available to accomplish body functions
  - **Adipose tissue** Ⓘ is burned to produce energy
  - **Body temperature** Ⓙ increases, because heat is produced as a byproduct of metabolic reactions

Regulation of Thyroid Hormones

- T_4, T_3 synthesis stimulated by **thyroid stimulating hormone** Ⓚ (TSH, from **pituitary gland** Ⓛ)
- TSH synthesis stimulated by **thyrotropin releasing hormone** (TRH Ⓜ, from the **hypothalamus** Ⓝ)
- TRH secretion stimulated by **stress and cold** Ⓞ, inhibited by heat
- T_4 and T_3 inhibit the production of TSH and TRH
  - **Negative feedback** Ⓟ
  - Maintains thyroid hormone concentrations within normal limits

Thyroid Hormone Dysfunction

Disorder	Cause	Some Symptoms
Hyperthyroidism Ⓠ (excess thyroid hormone)	Abnormal stimulation of thyroid gland (Grave's disease), thyroid tumor	Heat intolerance, weight loss, anxiety, rapid heart rate, exophthalmos (bulgy eyes), large thyroid (goiter)
Hypothyroidism Ⓡ (insufficient thyroid hormone)	Thyroid atrophy, pituitary failure	Cold intolerance, weight gain, slow thought, slow heart rate, swollen face, normal or small thyroid

A. thyroid hormone
B. thyroid gland
C. growth
D. brain development
E. heart rate
F. brain activity
G. nutrients
H. energy
 I. adipose
J. body temperature
K. TSH
L. anterior pituitary
   gland
M. TRH
N. hypothalamus
O. cold, stress
 P. negative feedback
Q. hyperthyroidism
R. hypothyroidism

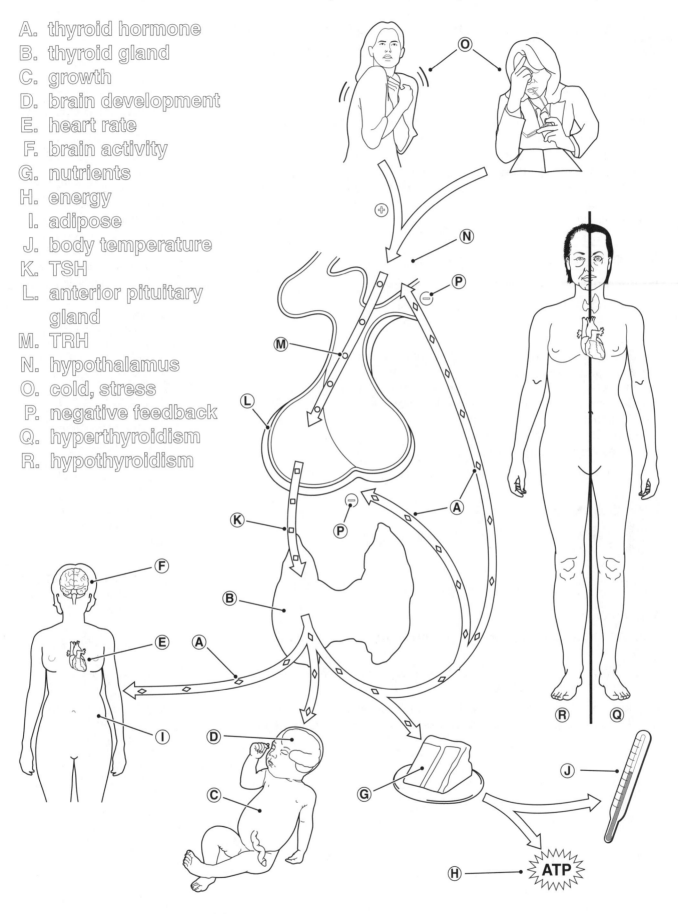

Coloring Exercise 7-7 ➤ Adrenal Hormones: Epinephrine and Aldosterone

Adrenal Gland

- Inner **medulla** (A), synthesizes **norepinephrine** and **epinephrine** (B)
- Outer **cortex** (C), synthesizes adrenal steroids
  - Mineralocorticoids (**aldosterone** (D)): regulate salt balance (see below)
  - Glucocorticoids (**cortisol** (E)): important in the stress response (for instance, starvation on a desert island; see Coloring Exercise 7-8)
  - **Sex steroids** (F): induce male characteristics in females (facial hair, etc.); minimal effects in males

Norepinephrine and Epinephrine

- Closely related hormones
- Help body respond to emergency situations
- Effects include
  - **Pupil** dilation (G)
  - Dilation of **airways** (H), to permit deeper breaths
  - Increased **blood pressure** (I) and **heart rate** (J)
  - Increased conversion of glycogen into glucose in the **liver** (K)
  - Decreased activity of **gastrointestinal tract** (L)
  - Dilation of blood vessels in **muscle** (M)
  - Contraction of the **bladder** (N)
  - Increased metabolic rate of cells
- Secreted when the sympathetic nervous system is activated

Aldosterone (D)

- Acts at **kidney** (O) to increase **sodium** (Na) (P) retention and decrease **potassium** (K) (Q) retention
  - Less Na leaves body in **urine** (R); **blood** (S) Na concentrations increase
  - More K leaves body in urine; blood K concentrations decrease

Regulation

- Secretion stimulated by high plasma **potassium** (Q), inhibited by low plasma potassium
- Low plasma sodium levels stimulate release indirectly, via the renin-angiotensin system (**RAAS**) (T)
- Aldosterone increases blood Na levels and decreases blood K levels
  - These changes reduce aldosterone secretion by **negative feedback** (U)

COLORING INSTRUCTIONS

Color each figure part and its name at the same time, using the same color. Save light red, dark red, green, brown, and yellow for later.

1. Color the adrenal medulla (A) and cortex (C).
2. Color the arrows representing the different adrenal hormones ((B), (D) to (F)) and the cartoons reflecting their actions.
3. On the middle figure, color the different organs affected by norepinephrine/epinephrine ((G) to (N)).

COLORING INSTRUCTIONS

On the bottom left figure:

1. Color the kidney (O) brown, the urine (R) light yellow, and the blood vessel (S) light red.
2. Color the letters indicating sodium (Na (P)) and potassium (K (Q)).

COLORING INSTRUCTIONS

On the bottom right figure:

1. Color the adrenal cortex (C) and the kidney (O).
2. Color the large arrow leaving the adrenal cortex, representing aldosterone (D).
3. Color the letters indicating sodium (Na (P)) and potassium (K (Q)), and the renin-angiotensin system (RAAS (T)).
4. Color the negative signs, representing negative feedback (U).

A. adrenal medulla
B. epinephrine/ norepinephrine
C. adrenal cortex
D. aldosterone
E. cortisol
F. sex steroids
G. pupil
H. airways
I. blood pressure
J. heart rate
K. liver
L. gastrointestinal tract
M. muscle
N. bladder
O. kidney
P. sodium (Na)
Q. potassium (K)
R. urine
S. blood
T. RAAS
U. negative feedback

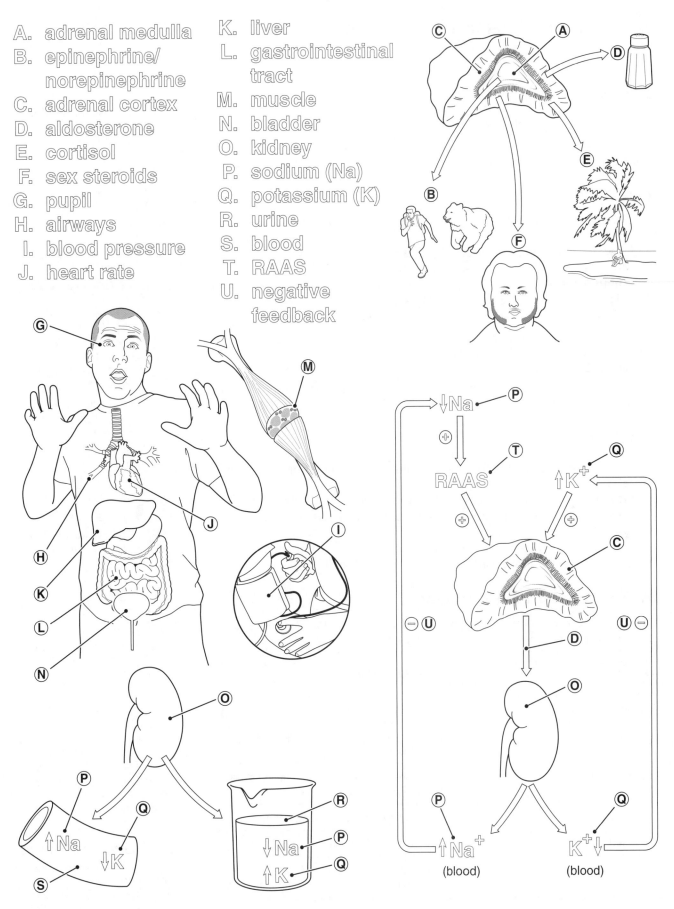

Coloring Exercise 7-8 ➤ Adrenal Hormones: Glucocorticoids

Cortisol Ⓐ

- Synthesized in adrenal cortex
- Helps body respond to stress by increasing available nutrients for energy and tissue repair

Roles

- Storage forms of nutrients are converted into readily available forms and secreted into blood
  - **Liver** Ⓑ: **glycogen** Ⓒ converted to **glucose** Ⓓ
  - **Muscle** Ⓔ and connective tissue (not shown): **protein** Ⓕ converted to **amino acids** Ⓖ
  - **Adipose** Ⓗ: **fat** Ⓘ converted to **fatty acids** Ⓙ
- Nutrients used to
  - Generate glucose from amino acids (gluconeogenesis)
  - Provide **energy** Ⓚ (all nutrients)
  - **Repair tissues** Ⓛ (amino acids)
- Inhibits the inflammatory response and immune system in high doses (medicinal use)

Regulation

- Secretion regulated by the hypothalamopituitary axis and **negative feedback** Ⓜ
  - **Pituitary** Ⓝ adrenocorticotropin (**ACTH** Ⓞ) induces cortisol release
  - **Hypothalamic** Ⓟ corticotrophin releasing hormone (**CRH** Ⓠ) induces ACTH release
  - CRH release stimulated by physical (starvation, trauma or emotional stress)
  - Cortisol from **adrenal gland** Ⓢ inhibits CRH and ACTH release

Dysfunction: Cushing Syndrome

Cushing syndrome Ⓣ caused by excess activity of the pituitary or adrenal gland or overmedication with corticosteroids

Symptom or Sign	Explanation
Thinning extremities, muscle wasting and weakness	Cortisol stimulates muscle breakdown
High blood sugar	Cortisol stimulates glycogen breakdown, gluconeogenesis
Easy bruising	Cortisol stimulates connective tissue breakdown
Poor healing	Cortisol inhibits immune function
Increased facial hair	(actions of adrenal sex steroids)
Truncal obesity	High blood sugar stimulates insulin production, insulin stimulates fat deposition

---

COLORING INSTRUCTIONS

Color each figure part and its name at the same time, using the same color. On the top figure:

1. Lightly color the organs targeted by cortisol: (liver Ⓑ, muscle Ⓔ, and adipose Ⓗ).
2. Color the nutrients wherever they are found (blood and tissues). Use related colors for glucose Ⓓ and glycogen Ⓒ, amino acids Ⓖ and proteins Ⓕ, and fatty acids Ⓙ and fats Ⓘ. Use the same colors as in Coloring Exercise 7-3.
4. Color the arrows Ⓐ, representing metabolic actions of cortisol.
5. Color the injured tissue Ⓛ and the ATP molecule Ⓚ, representing uses for the nutrients.

COLORING INSTRUCTIONS

On the bottom left figure:

1. Color the hypothalamus Ⓟ and CRH molecules Ⓠ leaving the hypothalamus.
2. Color the anterior pituitary gland Ⓝ and ACTH molecules Ⓞ leaving the pituitary.
3. Color the adrenal cortex Ⓣ and cortisol molecules Ⓐ, traveling to the anterior pituitary gland and hypothalamus to inhibit their activity. Color the negative signs Ⓜ representing negative feedback.

COLORING INSTRUCTIONS

On the bottom right, color the cartoon illustrating the symptoms of Cushing syndrome Ⓤ. Use this cartoon to remind yourself of the effects of glucocorticoids.

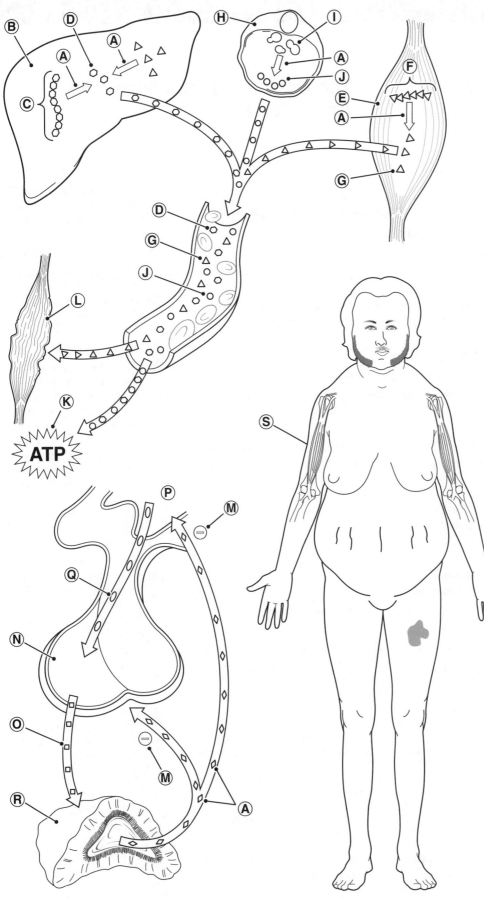

A. cortisol
B. liver
C. glycogen
D. glucose
E. muscle
F. protein
G. amino acids
H. adipose
I. fat
J. fatty acids
K. energy
L. tissue repair
M. negative
   feedback
N. pituitary gland
O. ACTH
P. hypothalamus
Q. CRH
R. adrenal gland
S. Cushing
   syndrome

ATP

CHAPTER 8

The Cardiovascular System

Coloring Exercise 8-1 ➤ The Cardiovascular System: An Overview

Components

- Blood (Coloring Exercises 8-3 to 8-5): the fluid of life, carrying substances to cells (oxygen, nutrients) and away from cells (carbon dioxide, waste products)
- Blood vessels: pathways for blood movement
- Heart: propels blood through blood vessels

Heart

- The **heart** (A) (Coloring Exercises 8-6 to 8-8) is a fist-shaped, muscular organ located in between **right** (B) and **left** (C) **lungs**, above the **diaphragm** (D)
  - Upper **base** (A1), lower **apex** (A2)
  - Protected by bony cage of **ribs** (E)
- Surrounded by connective tissue sac (the **pericardium** (F))
- Cardiac muscle (Coloring Exercise 4-1) provides force that propels blood

Blood Vessels

- Blood vessels (Coloring Exercises 8-9 to 8-16) contain up to three tissue types, which may be separated by layers of **elastic tissue** (G)
  - **Inner tunic: endothelium** (H)
    - Squamous (flat) epithelial cells (Coloring Exercise 1-7)
    - Provides smooth surface for blood flow
  - **Middle tunic: smooth muscle** (I)
    - Contracts to shrink vessel diameter
    - Controlled by autonomic nervous system
  - **Outer tunic: connective tissue** (J)
    - Strengthens and supports blood vessel
- Blood leaving the **heart** (A) passes through different types of vessels, listed below in order

	Structure	Function
1. **Arteries** (K)	Thick outer tunic Two smooth muscle layers Extensive elastic tissue	Carry blood from heart; resist strong forces created by heart
2. **Arterioles** (L)	(not shown) Thinner walls than arteries; lots of smooth muscle	Change diameter to regulate blood pressure; convey blood to capillaries
3. **Capillaries** (M)	Only endothelium	Sites of gas exchange
4. **Venules** (N)	Contain progressively larger amounts of the outer tunics	Formed by merging capillaries; convey blood to veins
5. **Veins** (O)	Contain all tunics and **valves** (P); thin muscle layer	Return blood to heart; valves prevent blood backflow away from heart

✎ **COLORING INSTRUCTIONS**
Color each structure and its name at the same time, using the same color.

1. Color all of the labeled parts ((A) to (F)). Do not use red, blue, or purple.
2. Use the same color for (A), (A1), and (A2).
3. Use a dark color to outline the pericardium (F).
4. On the bottom figure, begin with the heart on the far left (A). As you move left to right, color the different vessel types ((K) to (O)). Use the following color scheme: arteries (K) red, arterioles (L) light red, capillaries (M) purple, venules (N) light blue, veins (O) dark blue. Note that there are many more branchings than are shown here.
5. As you read through the table, color the different tunics in each vessel type ((H) to (J)) in the middle figure. Note that capillaries (at the bottom of the diagram) are composed solely of endothelium (H).
6. Color the valves (P) in the vein by lightly shading over the tunics you colored in step 2.

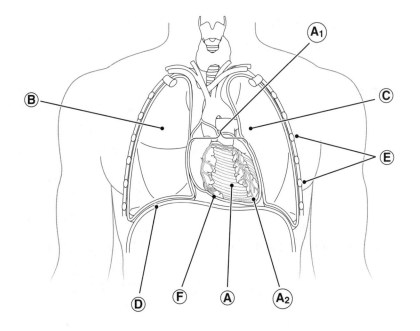

A. heart
A₁. base
A₂. apex
B. right lung
C. left lung
D. diaphragm
E. ribs
F. pericardium

G. elastic tissue
H. inner tunic: endothelium
I. middle tunic: smooth muscle
J. outer tunic: connective tissue
K. arteries

L. arterioles
M. capillaries
N. venules
O. veins
P. valves

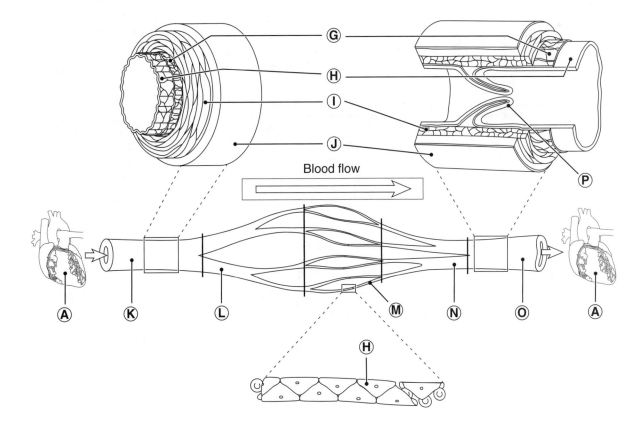

Coloring Exercise 8-2 ➤ The Pulmonary and Systemic Circulations

Pulmonary Circulation: Gas Exchange

- Involves the right side of the heart
- Carbon dioxide moves from blood to lungs, oxygen from lungs to blood
- Blood arriving in lungs is relatively low in oxygen (deoxygenated)
  - Blood is bluish in color
- Blood leaving the lungs is relatively high in oxygen
  - Blood is redder in color

Systemic Circulation: Nourishment and Waste Removal

- Involves the left side of the heart
- All tissues (including the heart) receive oxygenated blood from the left side of the heart
- Tissues remove oxygen, add carbon dioxide

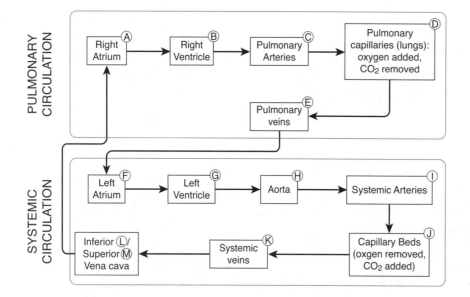

✏️ **COLORING INSTRUCTIONS**

Color each structure and its corresponding term at the same time, using the same color. Read all instructions before beginning this Coloring Exercise.

1. Use the following color scheme:

   Pulmonary Ⓓ and systemic Ⓙ capillary beds: variants of purple.

   Systemic arteries Ⓘ and pulmonary veins Ⓔ: variants of red (could also use pink and orange if necessary).

   Systemic veins Ⓚ and pulmonary arteries Ⓒ: variants of blue.

2. Start with the pulmonary circulation (top part of the flowchart). Follow the blood through the pulmonary circulation, starting with the right atrium Ⓐ. Color the structures on the right-hand page and lightly shade the flowchart boxes on the left-hand page as you go. If you wish, draw arrows to indicate the direction of blood flow on the diagram.

3. Repeat step two for the systemic circulation, beginning with the left atrium.

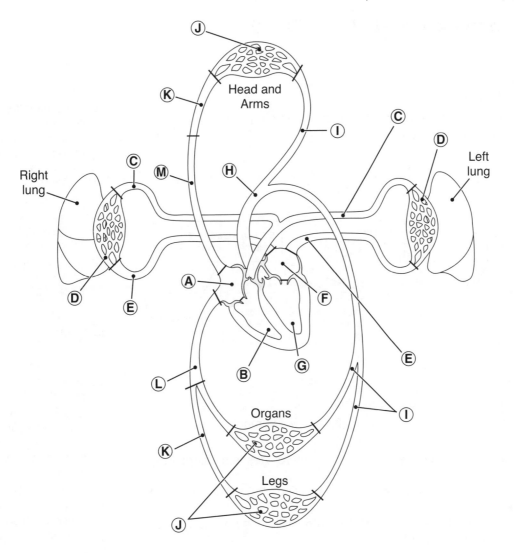

A. right atrium
B. right ventricle
C. pulmonary arteries
D. pulmonary capillaries
E. pulmonary veins
F. left atrium
G. left ventricle

H. aorta
I. systemic arteries
J. capillary beds
K. systemic veins
L. inferior vena cava
M. superior vena cava

Coloring Exercise 8-3 ➤ Blood

Blood Constituents

- **Blood** (A) can be separated into components by centrifugation
- Heavier elements sink to the bottom of the tube

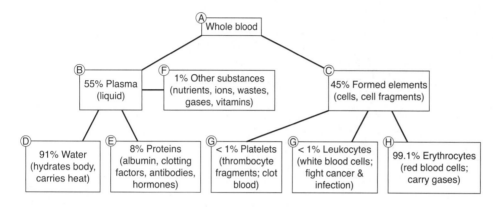

Hematocrit

- Volume percentage of erythrocytes in whole blood
- Normal hematocrit: 42%–54% (men) or 36%–46% (women)
- **Anemia** (H1): low hematocrit (too few erythrocytes)
  - Hemolytic anemia: abnormal destruction of erythrocytes (e.g., sickle-cell anemia)
  - Deficiency anemia: insufficient erythrocyte building blocks (such as iron or vitamin B12)
  - Aplastic anemia: insufficient erythrocyte synthesis in bone marrow, reflecting bone marrow damage or cancer
- **Polycythemia** (H2): high hematocrit
  - Too many erythrocytes: bone marrow disorder, living at high altitude
  - Insufficient plasma: dehydration

Regulation of Erythrocyte Synthesis

1. Blood **oxygen** (I) levels drop
2. Low blood oxygen stimulates **erythropoietin** (J) synthesis by kidney (K)
3. Erythropoietin stimulates **erythrocyte** (H) synthesis by the **bone marrow** (L)
4. Erythrocytes carry more oxygen in the blood
5. Blood oxygen levels increase; the stimulus for erythropoietin secretion is removed

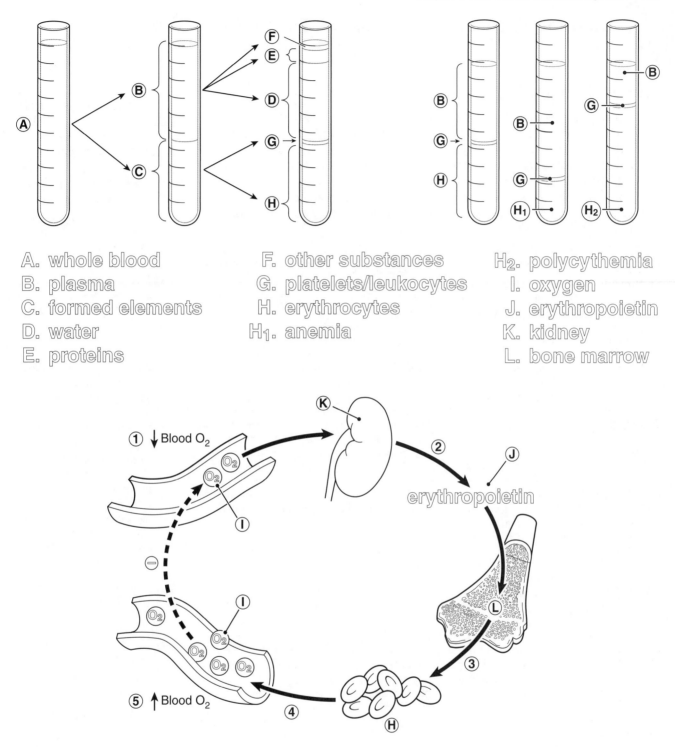

A. whole blood
B. plasma
C. formed elements
D. water
E. proteins

F. other substances
G. platelets/leukocytes
H. erythrocytes
H₁. anemia

H₂. polycythemia
I. oxygen
J. erythropoietin
K. kidney
L. bone marrow

Coloring Exercise 8-4 ➤ Blood: Formed Elements

Formed Elements

- Blood cells can be identified in blood smears
  - Blood droplet placed on microscope slide and "smeared" to produce a thin film
  - Smears usually stained with Wright's stain to visualize nuclei, granules, and cytoplasm
  - Differential blood count: identifies the number of each white blood cell (WBC) type in one microliter of blood: elevations or decreases can indicate disease

Cell Type	Appearance*	Function	Changes in Disease
Erythrocyte Ⓐ	Pink, no nucleus or granules; packed with **hemoglobin** Ⓐ1	Carries oxygen, carbon dioxide, hydrogen ions	See Coloring Exercise 8-2
Neutrophil Ⓑ (54%–62% of WBCs)	Nucleus: lobed, dark purple Granules: fine, not usually visible Cytoplasm: pale pink	Phagocytosis of bacteria, other invaders	↑: infection, arthritis, some cancers, physical stress
Eosinophil Ⓒ (1%–3% of WBCs)	Nucleus: purple Granules: large, bright pink Cytoplasm: pale pink	Fight parasites, may inhibit allergic responses	↑: allergic events, drug reactions, parasitic infection, some malignancies
Lymphocyte Ⓓ (25%–38% of WBCs)	Nucleus: deep purple Granules: few if any Cytoplasm: blue	Involved in specific immune responses	↑: acute infection, lymphoid malignancy ↓: AIDS
Basophil Ⓔ (1% of WBCs)	Nucleus: dark blue, often obscured by granules Granules: large, dark blue Cytoplasm: pink	May mediate allergic responses	↑: Rare, may indicate viral infections, inflammation
Monocyte Ⓕ (3%–7% of WBCs)	Nucleus: purple Granules: few if any Cytoplasm: light blue	Precursor to macrophage (macrophages phagocytose microbes)	↑: infection (usually bacterial)
Platelets Ⓖ	Granules: purple Cytoplasm: light blue	Blood clotting	↓: cancer treatment, leukemia, some cancers

*Appearance after staining with Wright's stain

COLORING INSTRUCTIONS

Color each structure and its corresponding term at the same time, using the same color.

1. Color a few erythrocytes Ⓐ bright red in each figure.

2. Color the hemoglobin molecule Ⓐ1 using a related color.

3. Color the names of the six other formed elements (Ⓑ to Ⓖ) using dark colors (not blue, pink, or purple). Use these colors to outline the box surrounding the relevant figure, and (if you like) the row of the table.

4. Use the colors listed in the table to color the nucleus, granules, and cytoplam of the different blood cells. For instance, color the eosinophil nucleus purple, the cytoplasm pale pink, and the granules dark pink (Ⓒ).

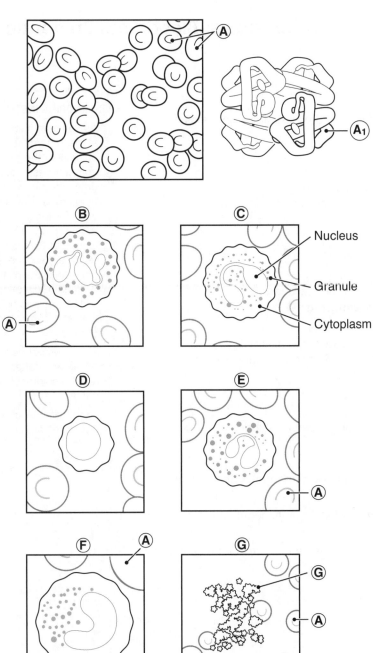

A. erythrocyte
A_1. hemoglobin
B. neutrophil
C. eosinophil
D. lymphocyte
E. basophil
F. monocyte
G. platelets

Nucleus

Granule

Cytoplasm

Coloring Exercise 8-5 ➤ Hemostasis: Blood Loss Prevention

Hemostasis

- Process that prevents loss of **blood cells** Ⓐ and plasma following **vessel injury** Ⓑ
- Vessel wall components include:
  - **Endothelium** Ⓒ: inner epithelial lining
  - **Smooth muscle** Ⓓ: determines vessel diameter
  - Extracellular matrix (especially **collagen** Ⓔ): surrounds blood vessel
- First stage: **Vasoconstriction** Ⓕ
  - Vascular **smooth muscle** Ⓓ contracts
  - Vessel diameter shrinks, limiting blood loss
- Second stage: Platelet plug formation
  - **Platelets** Ⓖ, other blood components contact collagen
  - Platelets become sticky, forming a **platelet plug** Ⓖ⚊
- Third stage: Coagulation (clotting) and hemostasis
  - **Fibrinogen** Ⓗ: soluble plasma protein (dissolved in plasma)
  - Fibrinogen converts to **fibrin** Ⓘ, which forms solid threads
  - Fibrin strands and red blood cells form a clot

Control of Blood Clot Formation

- Multi-step pathway controls conversion of fibrinogen into fibrin
- Initiated by two stimuli
  - Exposed **collagen** Ⓔ
  - **Tissue factor** Ⓙ: membrane receptor made by damaged endothelial cells (and other cells)
- Many other factors stimulate (coagulants) or inhibit (anticoagulants) the clotting pathway
- Factor (thrombin) that activates clot formation also stimulates clot dissolution by activating **plasmin** Ⓚ

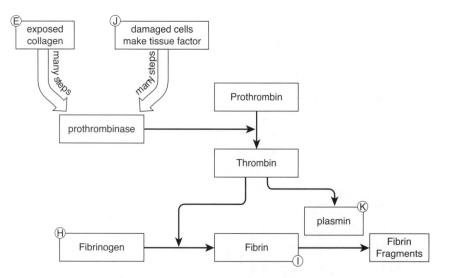

A. blood cells
B. injury
C. endothelium
D. smooth muscle
E. collagen
F. vasoconstriction
G. platelets
G₁. platelet plug
H. fibrinogen
I. fibrin
J. tissue factor
K. plasmin

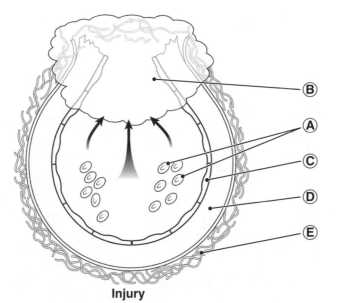

Injury

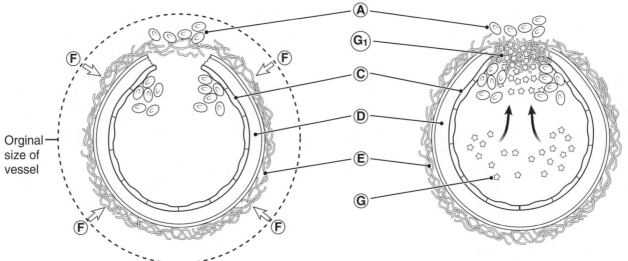

Orginal size of vessel

Vasoconstriction

Platelet plug formation

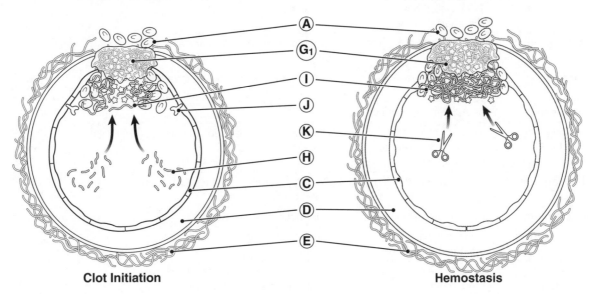

Clot Initiation

Hemostasis

Coloring Exercise 8-6 ➤ Anatomy of the Heart

Name	Structure	Function
Superior vena cava Ⓐ	Large vein	Delivers deoxygenated blood from above diaphragm to heart
Inferior vena cava Ⓑ	Large vein	Delivers deoxygenated blood from lower body to heart
Right atrium Ⓒ	Thin-walled heart chamber; upper right	Receives blood from venae cavae and coronary sinus (Coloring Exercise 8-7)
Right AV valve Ⓓ	Valve separating right atrium and ventricle; three cusps	Prevents backflow of blood from the ventricle to the atrium
Right ventricle Ⓔ	Thin-walled heart chamber (thicker than atria); lower right	Receives blood from right atrium, delivers it to pulmonary trunk
Pulmonary valve Ⓕ	Three-cusp valve at pulmonary trunk entrance	Prevents backflow from pulmonary artery into right ventricle
Pulmonary trunk Ⓖ	Large artery	Delivers blood to pulmonary arteries
Right Ⓗ, left Ⓘ pulmonary arteries	The only arteries carrying deoxygenated blood	Deliver deoxygenated blood to lungs
Right Ⓙ, left Ⓚ lungs	Site of gas exchange between air and blood	Add oxygen to blood, remove carbon dioxide from blood
Right Ⓛ, left Ⓜ pulmonary veins	The only veins carrying oxygenated blood	Deliver oxygenated blood to left atrium
Left atrium Ⓝ	Thin-walled heart chamber; upper left	Receives blood from pulmonary veins, delivers it to left ventricle
Left AV valve Ⓞ	Valve separating left atrium and ventricle; two cusps	Prevents backflow of blood from the ventricle to the atrium
Left ventricle Ⓟ	Thick-walled heart chamber; lower left	Receives blood from left atrium; delivers it to aorta
Aortic valve Ⓠ	Valve at aorta entrance; three cusps	Prevents backflow from aorta into left ventricle
Aorta Ⓡ	Thick-walled artery	Delivers oxygenated blood to body
Chordae tendineae Ⓢ	Tendons connecting papillary muscle and valves	Prevent valves from turning inside out
Papillary muscle Ⓣ	Muscles connecting chordae tendineae to heart muscle	Help chordae tendineae keep valves in place
Endocardium Ⓤ	Innermost heart lining; epithelial tissue	Provides a smooth surface to prevent blood clotting
Myocardium Ⓥ	Cardiac muscle	Contracts to propel blood
Epicardium Ⓦ	Connective tissue (serous membrane)	Protects myocardium; forms serous pericardium
Fibrous pericardium (not shown)	Thick connective tissue membrane	Protects and encloses heart; space between fibrous and serous pericardium can become infected

✎ COLORING INSTRUCTIONS

1. As you read through the table, color the different heart structures and the corresponding terms. Color the table row with the same color if you wish.

2. For the endocardium Ⓤ, just color this heart wall layer in cross section (the narrow line). The entire interior of the heart that is visible is actually endocardium.

3. If you wish, draw arrows to represent the flow of blood through the heart. Use blue arrows for deoxygenated blood and red arrows for oxygenated blood. The pathway of blood flow is shown in the flowchart of Coloring Exercise 8-2.

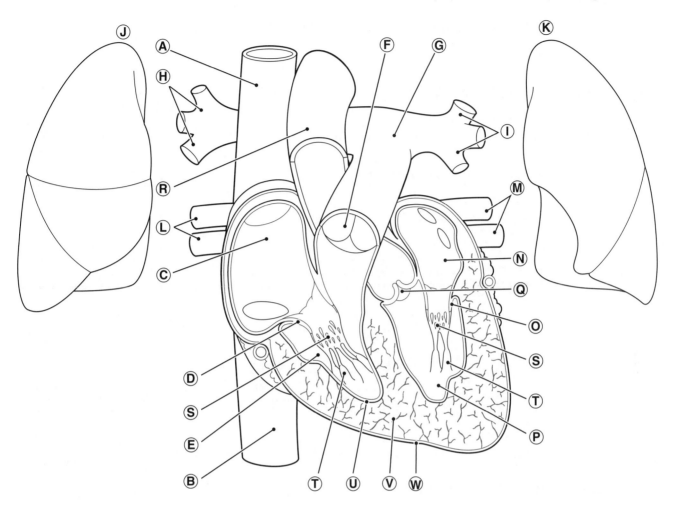

A. superior vena cava
B. inferior vena cava
C. right atrium
D. right AV valve
E. right ventricle
F. pulmonary valve
G. pulmonary trunk
H. right pulmonary arteries
I. left pulmonary arteries
J. right lung
K. left lung
L. right pulmonary vein

M. left pulmonary vein
N. left atrium
O. left AV valve
P. left ventricle
Q. aortic valve
R. aorta
S. chordae tendineae
T. papillary muscle
U. endocardium
V. myocardium
W. epicardium

Coloring Exercise 8-7 ➤ The Cardiac Vessels

Arterial Supply to the Heart Muscle

- The flowchart below illustrates blood flow through the coronary arteries
- All cardiac arteries send smaller branches to nourish the heart muscle
- Anastomosis: communication between two arteries
  - If one artery is blocked, the blood can travel through the other artery

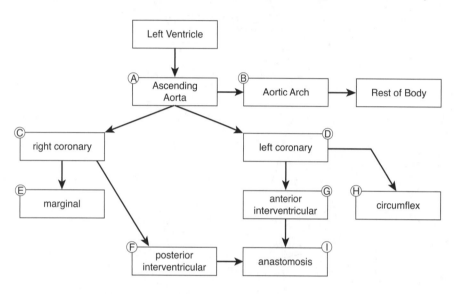

Venous Drainage of the Heart Muscle

- Blood from the walls of the right atrium and ventricle drains into the anterior cardiac veins
- Blood from the walls of the left atrium and ventricle eventually drains in the coronary sinus (sinus: large channel draining deoxygenated blood)
- The flowchart below illustrates the patterns of blood flow through the coronary veins.

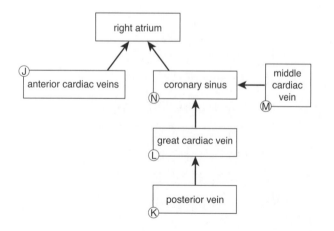

✎ **COLORING INSTRUCTIONS**

Color each structure and its corresponding term at the same time, using the same color.

1. The locations of the ventricles and atria are labeled for orientation purposes. Remember that these structures are chambers within the heart, not structures on the outside of the heart.

2. Use red-related colors for the arteries (such as reds, pinks, and oranges).

3. Go through the flow chart and both views (anterior/posterior) together, following the blood as it leaves the left ventricle.

4. Color the vessels, and lightly shade (or outline) the flowchart boxes, in alphabetical order (Ⓐ to Ⓗ).

5. Outline the circle surrounding the anastomosis Ⓘ between the posterior and anterior interventricular arteries.

6. Color all of the offshoots (arterioles) of the arteries the same color as the supplying artery.

✎ **COLORING INSTRUCTIONS**

1. Use variants of blue and purple to color the veins.

2. Go through the flow chart and the figures together, following the blood draining from different heart muscle regions to enter the right atrium.

3. Color the vessels, and lightly shade (or outline) the flowchart boxes, in alphabetical order (Ⓙ to Ⓝ).

4. Color the venules the same color as the vein into which they drain.

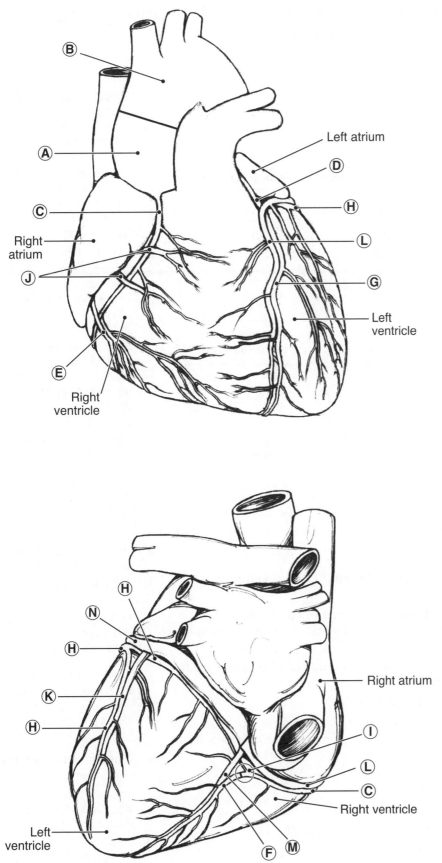

A. ascending aorta
B. aortic arch
C. right coronary artery
D. left coronary artery
E. marginal artery
F. posterior interventricular artery
G. anterior interventricular artery
H. circumflex artery
I. anastomosis
J. anterior cardiac veins
K. posterior vein
L. great cardiac vein
M. middle cardiac vein
N. coronary sinus

Left atrium

Right atrium

Right ventricle

Left ventricle

Right atrium

Right ventricle

Left ventricle

Coloring Exercise 8-8 ➤ The Cardiac Cycle and Conducting System

Cardiac Cycle

- Events that occur during one heart beat
- Diastole = relaxation
- Systole = contraction

	Diastole	Atrial Systole	Ventricular Systole
Atrial contraction Ⓐ?	No	Yes	No
Ventricular contraction Ⓑ?	No	No	Yes
Right Ⓒ **and left** Ⓓ **AV valves** open?	Yes	Yes	No
Pulmonary Ⓔ/**aortic** Ⓕ **valves** open?	No	No	Yes
Oxygenated Ⓖ **and de-oxygenated** Ⓗ **blood flow**?	Atria to ventricles	Atria to ventricles	Ventricles to aorta/pulmonary artery

Conduction System of the Heart

- Specialized muscle cells (conducting cells) convey signals
- Electrical signals stimulate nearby muscle cells to contract
- Sinoatrial node: initiates heart beat by generating action potentials
- Action potential spreads through conducting cells

Events

1. **Sinoatrial node** Ⓘ initiates action potential
   - Frequency of action potentials determines pulse
   - 72 action potentials/minute: pulse = 72
2. Action potential spreads through **atrial muscle cells** Ⓙ, causing the atria to contract (atrial systole).
3. Action potentials arrive at **atrioventricular (AV) node** Ⓚ, where there is a short delay. Action potentials cannot spread directly from atrial muscle cells to ventricle muscle cells.
4. Action potentials spread from AV node down the **bundle of His** Ⓛ, and down the right and left **bundle branches** Ⓛ①.
5. Action potentials spread through **Purkinje fibers** Ⓜ.
6. Purkinje fibers excite ventricular muscle cells (ventricular systole, not shown). The contraction begins at the bottom of the heart, squeezing blood upwards.

Electrocardiogram

- Record of the heart's electrical activity
- **P wave** Ⓝ: atrial depolarization
- **QRS wave** Ⓞ: ventricular depolarization (atrial repolarization)
- **T wave** Ⓟ: ventricular depolarization

✎ COLORING INSTRUCTIONS

Color each structure and its corresponding term at the same time, using the same color. On the top figure:

1. Color all of the elements of one diagram before proceeding to the next, beginning at the far left. Save red and blue.
2. Color the name of the stage in black.
3. Color the arrows representing contraction (if relevant) of the atria Ⓐ or the ventricles Ⓑ.
4. Color the valves (Ⓒ to Ⓕ). (They are only labeled on the first diagram.) Note if they are open or closed.
5. Color the arrows representing blood flow. Use red for oxygenated blood flow (left heart, Ⓖ) and blue for deoxygenated blood flow Ⓗ.

✎ COLORING INSTRUCTIONS

On the bottom left figure:

1. Color the elements of the cardiac conducting system.
2. The movement of action potentials through the atria (right heart, Ⓙ) is represented by arrows. Action potential conduction through the ventricles is not shown.

✎ COLORING INSTRUCTIONS

On the bottom right figure:

1. Color the three waveforms of the electrocardiogram.
2. Color the arrows representing atrial and ventricular contraction.

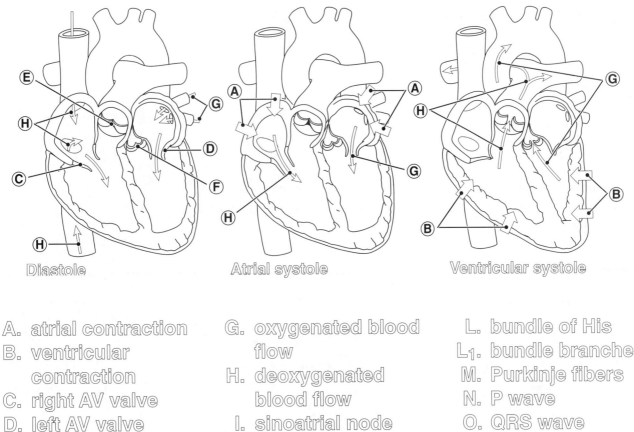

Diastole

Atrial systole

Ventricular systole

A. atrial contraction
B. ventricular contraction
C. right AV valve
D. left AV valve
E. pulmonary valve
F. aortic valve

G. oxygenated blood flow
H. deoxygenated blood flow
I. sinoatrial node
J. atrial muscle cells
K. atriovenricular node

L. bundle of His
L₁. bundle branches
M. Purkinje fibers
N. P wave
O. QRS wave
P. T wave

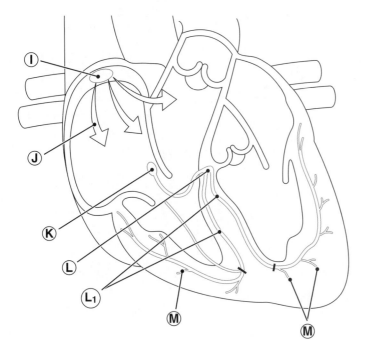

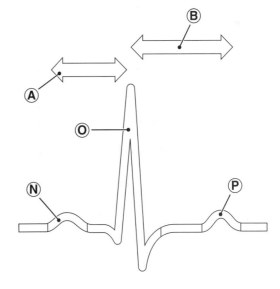

Coloring Exercise 8-9 ➤ Branches of the Aorta

Aorta

- Divided into four sections
  - **Ascending aorta** Ⓐ
  - **Aortic arch** Ⓑ
  - **Thoracic aorta** Ⓒ
  - **Abdominal aorta** Ⓓ, which branches into two **common iliac arteries** Ⓔ
- Each section has numerous branches supplying organs (dashed boxes, below) with oxygenated blood

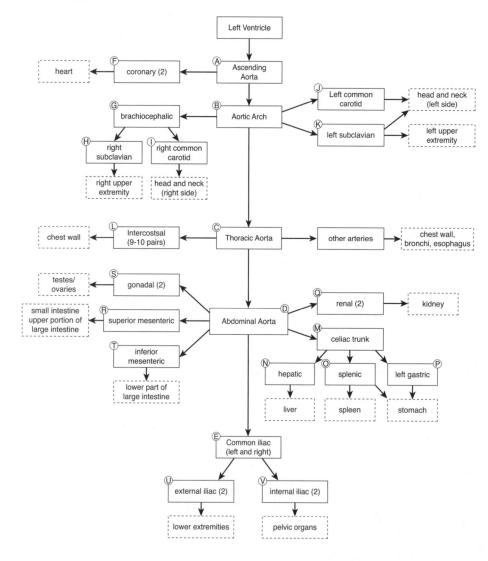

COLORING INSTRUCTIONS

1. Go through the flowchart and the figure together. Color the structure, the box in the flowchart, and the term with the same color.

2. Follow the path of the aorta (Ⓐ through Ⓓ) as it eventually splits into the two common iliac arteries Ⓔ.

3. Color the branches of the ascending aorta first, then the branches of the thoracic and abdominal aorta. Note that only one pair of intercostal arteries is labelled, and the celiac trunk Ⓜ is very short. Paired arteries are indicated by (2) after the name in the terms list.

4. Finally, color the branches of the common iliac arteries.

5. If you wish, color the organs using the same color as you used for the relevant artery. For instance, color the stomach with the color you used for the gastric artery.

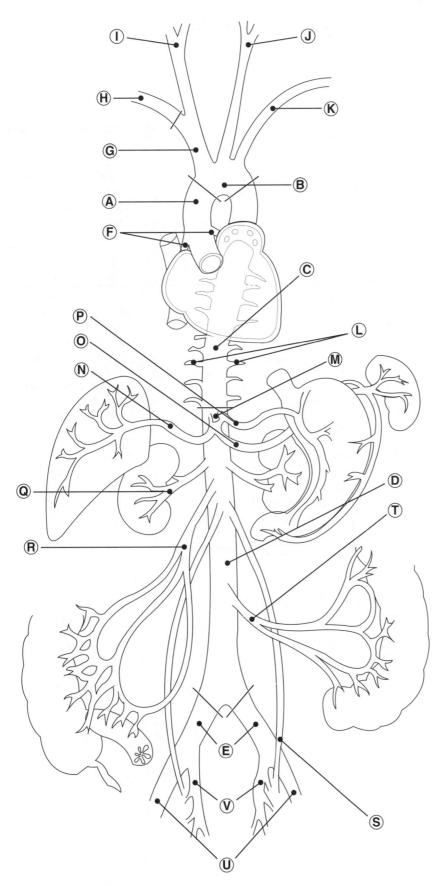

A. ascending aorta
B. aortic arch
C. thoracic aorta
D. abdominal aorta
E. common iliac (2)
F. coronary (2)
G. brachiocephalic
H. right subclavian
 I. right common
    carotid
J. left common
    carotid
K. left subclavian
L. intercostals (10
    pairs)
M. celiac trunk
N. hepatic
O. splenic
P. left gastric
Q. renal (2)
R. superior
    mesenteric
S. gonadal (2)
T. inferior
    mesenteric
U. external iliac (2)
V. internal iliac (2)

Coloring Exercise 8-10 ➤ Systemic Arteries

Systemic Arteries

- This Coloring Exercise shows the relationship between selected arteries of the upper extremity, neck, and lower limb.
- Arteries of the head: see Coloring Exercise 8-11
- Branches of the aorta: see Coloring Exercise 8-9
- Genicular artery is an anastomosis: junction of multiple arteries
  - Enables blood to bypass damage to one of the participating arteries

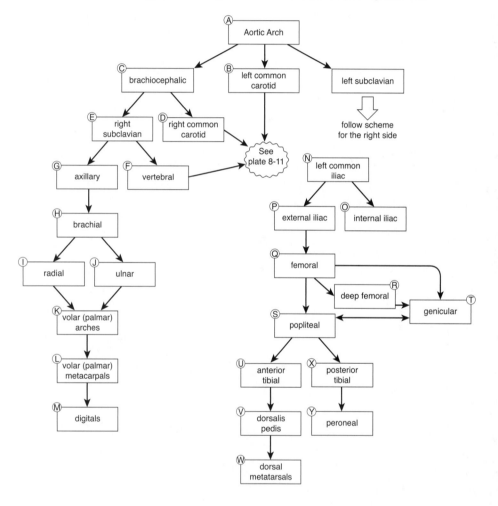

✍ **COLORING INSTRUCTIONS**

1. Go through the flowchart and the diagram, following the order of the letters. Lightly shade (or outline) the box on the flowchart, and the term in the list, with the same color used to color the artery.

2. Most arteries are paired—they occur on both sides of the body. Only one side is labeled for arteries Ⓕ to Ⓦ, but try to locate and color each artery on both sides of the body.

142

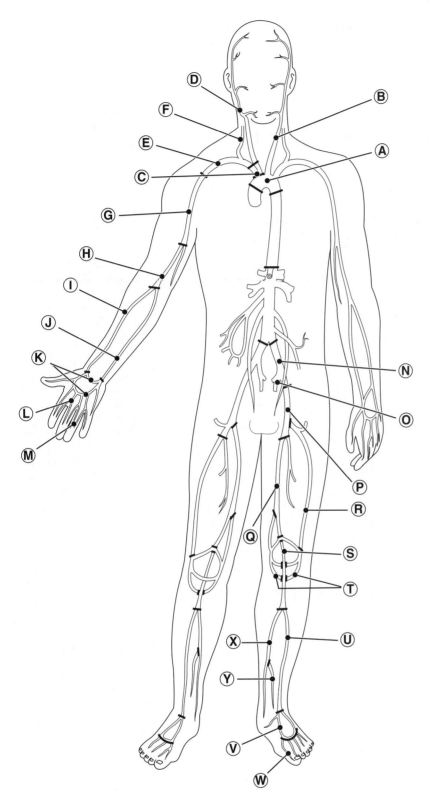

A. aortic arch
B. left common carotid
C. brachiocephalic
D. right comon carotid
E. right subclavian
F. vertebral
G. axillary
H. brachial
I. radial
J. ulnar
K. volar arches
L. volar metacarpals
M. digitals
N. left common iliac
O. internal iliac
P. external iliac
Q. femoral
R. deep femoral
S. popliteal
T. genicular
U. anterior tibial
V. dorsalis pedis
W. dorsal metatarsals
X. posterior tibial
Y. peroneal

Coloring Exercise 8-11 ➤ Arterial Supply to the Head

FLASHCARDS 35 AND 36

Arteries of the Face and Skull

- Branches of the **external carotid arteries** Ⓒ supply the face and skull
- The name of the artery describes the area it supplies

Arteries of the Brain: The Circle of Willis

- The **internal carotid** Ⓝ AND the **vertebral arteries** Ⓜ supply the brain
- Circle of Willis: large anastomosis supplied by the internal carotid and vertebral arteries
- Blockage to one artery does not completely block the brain's blood supply

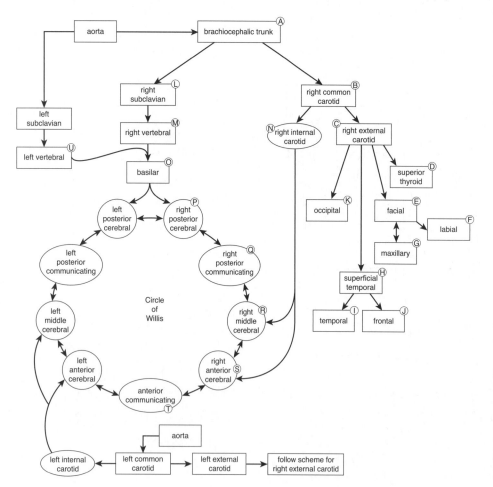

COLORING INSTRUCTIONS

On the top figure:

1. Follow blood travelling to the regions of the face and skull (Ⓐ to Ⓚ). Go through the flowchart and the diagram, following the order of the letters. Lightly shade (or outline) the box on the flowchart and the term in the list with the same color used to color the artery. Only the right side is shown.

On both figures:

2. Using the same procedure, follow blood travelling to the brain. Color arteries Ⓛ through Ⓜ on top figure, and arteries Ⓝ through Ⓣ on bottom figure. Only the arteries on the right side of the Circle of Willis are labelled. You can use the same color scheme to color the arteries of the left side.

3. Note that arteries making up the Circle of Willis are in circles, not boxes, in the flowchart.

4. Some vessels are described in the flowchart but not shown in the Figure. You can see these vessels on Figures 8-9 and 8-10.

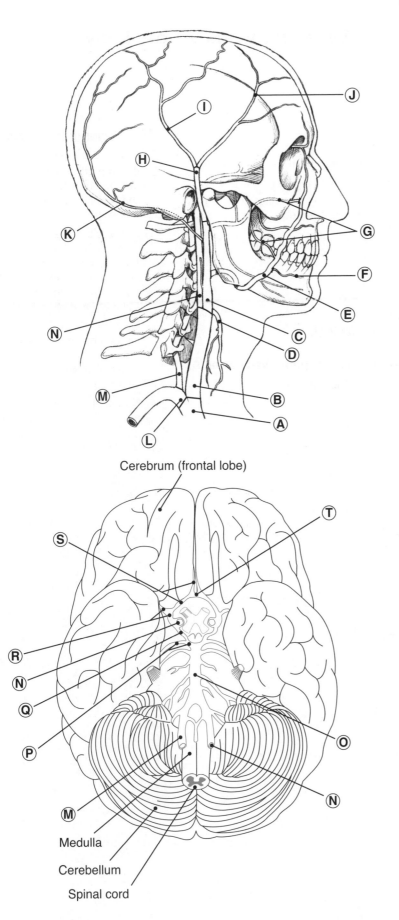

Cerebrum (frontal lobe)

Medulla

Cerebellum

Spinal cord

A. brachiocephalic trunk
B. right common carotid
C. right external carotid
D. superior thyroid
E. facial
F. labial
G. maxillary
H. superficial temporal
I. temporal
J. frontal
K. occipital
L. right subclavian
M. right vertebral
N. right internal carotid
O. basilar
P. right posterior cerebral
Q. right posterior communicating
R. right middle cerebral
S. right anterior cerebral
T. anterior communicating
U. left vertebral

Coloring Exercise 8-12 ➤ Systemic Veins: Upper Body

Veins: General Principles

- Two large veins return deoxygenated blood from body to heart
  - **Superior vena cava** Ⓓ: drains body above the diaphragm
  - Inferior vena cava: drains lower body (Coloring Exercise 8-13)
- Veins can be classified by location
  - Superficial veins: near body surface, often in extremities (e.g., Ⓔ)
  - Deep veins: often parallel arteries (e.g., Ⓐ)

Veins of the Upper Body

- Smaller veins merge to form larger veins, for instance:
  - **Brachial** Ⓚ + **basilic** Ⓘ = **axillary** Ⓛ
  - **Axillary** Ⓛ + **cephalic** Ⓗ = **subclavian** Ⓜ
  - **Subclavian** Ⓜ + **internal jugular** Ⓐ + **external jugular** Ⓑ = **brachiocephalic** Ⓒ
  - **Right brachiocephalic** Ⓒ + **left brachiocephalic** = **superior vena cava** Ⓓ
- Most veins are paired, but the **azygos vein** Ⓕ is unpaired

COLORING INSTRUCTIONS

1. Go through the flow-chart and the figure together. Some boxes list the regions drained by that vein.
2. Follow blood draining from the head (Ⓐ to Ⓓ), then from the chest wall (Ⓔ to Ⓕ), then from the upper limb (Ⓖ to Ⓜ). Color all hand veins Ⓖ the same color.
3. Lightly color or outline box with the same color as the term and the vein.
4. Note that only the right arm is shown.

A. internal jugular
B. external jugular
C. brachiocephalic
D. superior vena cava
E. intercostals
F. azygos
G. volar digitals
   and others
H. cephalic
 I. basilic
J. median cubital
K. brachial
L. axillary
M. subclavian

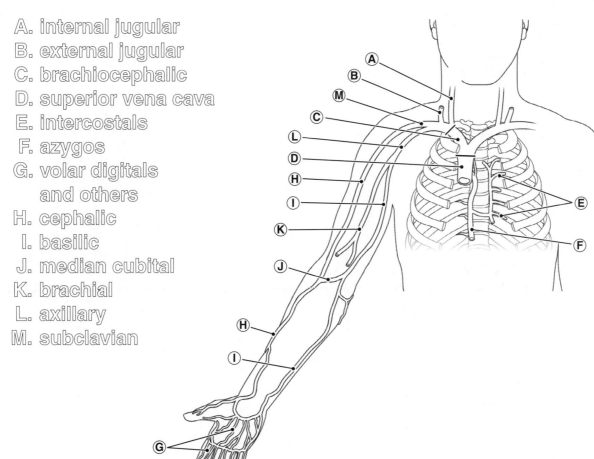

Coloring Exercise 8-13 ➤ Systemic Veins: Lower Body

FLASHCARDS 38 AND 39

Inferior Vena Cava

Inferior vena cava Ⓐ drains abdominal organs, pelvic organs, lower limb

Abdominal/Pelvic Veins

Hepatic vein Ⓑ receives blood from the hepatic portal circulation (drains gastrointestinal tract)

Veins of the Lower Limb

- Blood from lower limb drains into **external iliac vein** Ⓜ
- **Great saphenous vein** Ⓛ: longest vein in body; used for prolonged intravenous administration and for vessel grafts

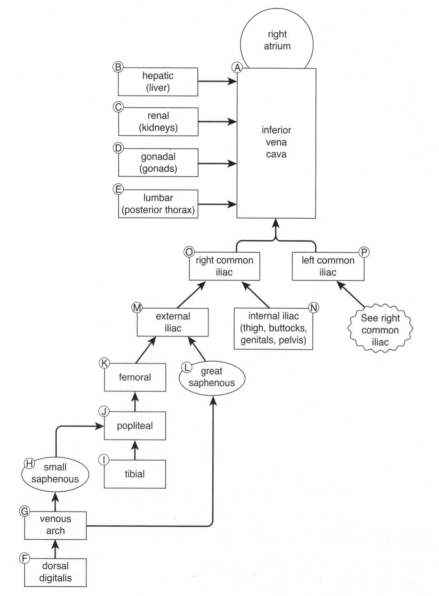

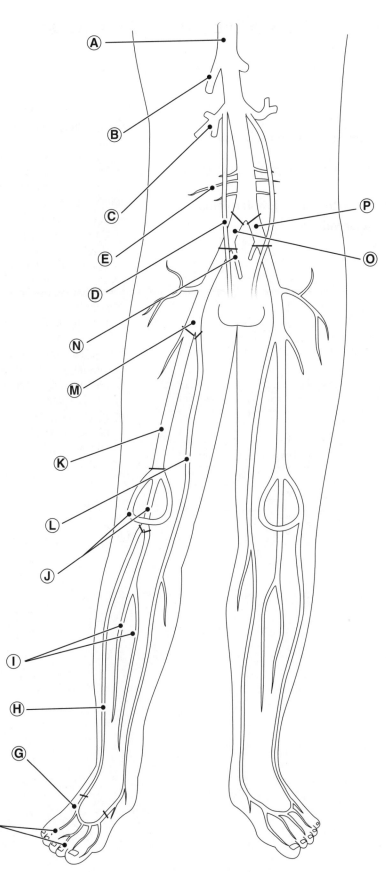

A. inferior vena cava
B. hepatic
C. renal
D. gonadal
E. lumbar
F. dorsal digitalis
G. venous arch
H. small saphenous
 I. tibial
J. popliteal
K. femoral
L. great saphenous
M. external iliac
N. internal iliac
O. right common
    iliac
P. left common
    iliac

Coloring Exercise 8-14 ➤ Venous Drainage of the Head

Veins and Sinuses

- All blood from brain drains into cranial venous sinuses, and subsequently into the **internal jugular veins** Ⓟ
  - Sinuses are large veins located between dura mater layers (see Coloring Exercise 5-7)
- Blood from face drains into **internal** Ⓟ and **external** Ⓑ **jugular veins**
- Blood from scalp drains into **external jugular vein** Ⓑ
- **Vertebral veins** Ⓕ drain neck structures

✎ **COLORING INSTRUCTIONS**

Note that only the right side is described. Only selected veins are labelled. Other veins (lightly shaded) are not to be colored.

1. Go through the flowchart and the diagram, following the order of the letters. Lightly shade (or outline) the box on the flowchart with the same color used to color the vein and the term.

2. Color the veins draining into the subclavian vein, and the right brachiocephalic vein (Ⓐ to Ⓕ).

3. Color the veins and sinuses draining into the internal jugular vein (Ⓖ to Ⓟ).

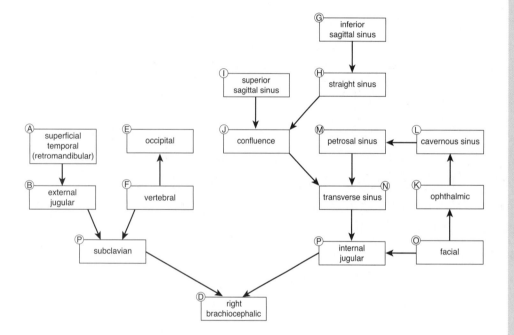

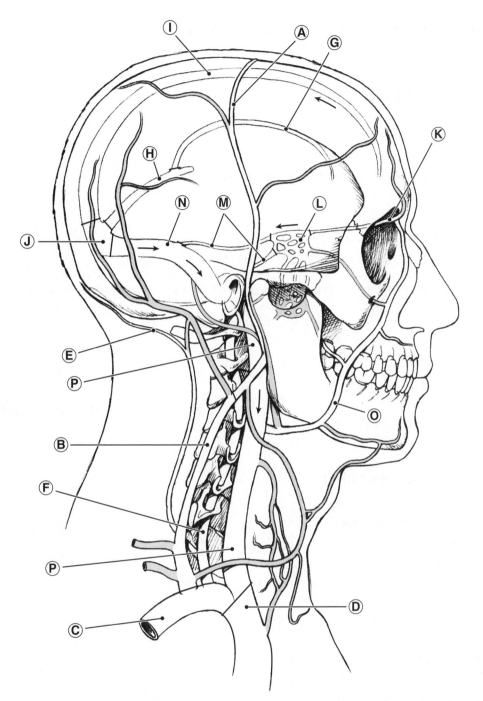

A. superficial temporal
B. external jugular
C. subclavian
D. right brachiocephalic
E. occipital
F. vertebral
G. inferior sagittal sinus
H. straight sinus

I. superior sagittal sinus
J. confluence
K. ophthalmic
L. cavernous sinus
M. petrosal sinuses
N. transverse sinus
O. facial
P. internal jugular

Coloring Exercise 8-15 ➤ Blood Pressure

Definition of Blood Pressure

Blood pressure Ⓐ:
- Provides force to push blood through the body
- Created by the heart, measured in the arteries
- Determined by **cardiac output** Ⓑ and **peripheral resistance** Ⓒ

Determinants

- Cardiac output = **stroke volume** Ⓓ x **heart rate** Ⓔ
  - Stroke volume = volume of blood ejected by heart in one heartbeat (stroke)
  - Sympathetic nervous system increases heart rate and stroke volume
- Peripheral resistance determined by
  - Vessel diameter (major determinant)
    - **Vasoconstriction** Ⓕ (constriction) increases blood pressure
    - **Vasodilation** Ⓖ (expansion) lowers blood pressure
    - Sympathetic nervous system causes overall vasoconstriction
  - **Total blood volume** Ⓗ
    - Higher volume increases blood pressure
  - **Blood viscosity** Ⓘ
    - Greater hematocrit reflects greater viscosity
    - Greater viscosity increases blood pressure

Control of Blood Pressure: Bleeding

1. An injury causes **bleeding** Ⓙ (hemorrhage)
2. Blood loss reduces **total blood volume** Ⓗ
3. **Peripheral resistance** Ⓒ is reduced.
4. **Blood pressure** Ⓐ drops.
5. **Baroreceptors** Ⓚ sense drop in blood pressure and send signal to brain.
6. **Brain** Ⓛ activates sympathetic nervous system.
7. Sympathetic nervous system induces:
   a. Increased **heart rate** Ⓔ
   b. Increased **stroke volume** Ⓓ
   c. Increased **vasoconstriction** Ⓕ
8. These changes raise blood pressure, partially compensating for blood loss.
9. Severe bleeding requires the administration of fluids (such as **intravenous fluids** Ⓜ) to restore blood volume and blood pressure to normal.

📝 **COLORING INSTRUCTIONS**

On the top figure:

1. As you proceed through the narrative, color the cartoons representing the determinants of blood pressure. For instance, a person pushing illustrates peripheral resistance.

2. Color each term in the list at the same time, using the corresponding color.

3. Use a dark color for Ⓔ to outline the ECG tracing, representing the heart rate.

📝 **COLORING INSTRUCTIONS**

On the bottom figure:

1. Go through the steps in the narrative and on the figure, beginning with step 1.

2. Color the labeled elements and the corresponding terms using the same color.

3. Color the arrows. Use green for up arrows (representing an increase) and red for down arrows (representing a decrease).

A. blood pressure
B. cardiac output
C. resistance

D. stroke volume
E. heart rate
F. vasoconstriction
G. vasodilation

H. total blood volume
I. blood viscosity
J. bleeding
K. baroreceptors
L. brain intravenous fluids

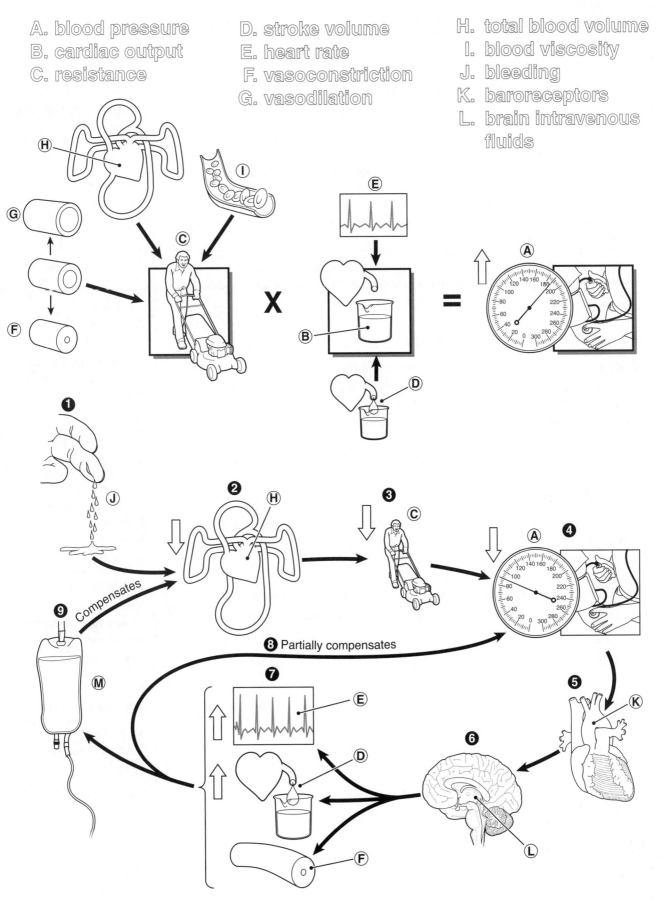

Coloring Exercise 8-16 ➤ Blood Flow: Capillary Beds and Veins

Blood Flow Through Capillary Beds

- Body does not contain enough blood to fill all vessels
- Blood flow to different organs controlled by altering **arteriole** Ⓑ diameter and by using **metarterioles** Ⓒ
  - Arteriole diameter controlled by contracting **smooth muscle** Ⓓ bands
    - Smooth muscle contraction, causing vasoconstriction, reduces blood available to the **capillary bed** Ⓐ
    - Smooth muscle relaxation, causing vasodilation, increases blood available to capillary bed
  - Blood travels through the capillary bed if the tissue needs blood, through the **metarteriole** Ⓒ if it does not (or other tissues need it more)
    - **Precapillary sphincter** Ⓔ contraction sends blood through the metarteriole
- Blood returns to the heart via **venules** Ⓕ and eventually veins (see below)

Gas Exchange in Capillary Beds

- **Capillary** walls Ⓐ are very thin to enable rapid diffusion
- In working tissues, **oxygen** Ⓖ diffuses from **red blood cells** Ⓗ, into the **interstitial fluid** Ⓘ, and finally into **tissue cells** Ⓙ
- **Carbon dioxide** Ⓚ diffuses in the other direction
- Nutrients (glucose, amino acids, lipids) and waste products, and other substances (not shown) are also exchanged between the capillary and the tissue

Venous Return

- Blood pressure is too low in **veins** Ⓛ (especially in the lower body) to propel blood back to heart
- **Skeletal muscle** Ⓜ contractions propel blood forward
- **Valves** Ⓝ prevent backflow of blood
  - Valves permit **blood flow** Ⓞ in only one direction (like a one-way door)
- Breathing (not shown) changes chest volume, sucking blood into the thorax

---

✐ **COLORING INSTRUCTIONS**

Color each structure and its corresponding term at the same time, using the same color. Beginning with the top left figure:

1. Color structures Ⓐ to Ⓕ in the larger diagram, but not in the magnification of the capillary.
2. Use variants of red for arterioles Ⓑ and metarterioles Ⓒ, use blue for venules Ⓕ, and purple for capillaries Ⓐ.

✐ **COLORING INSTRUCTIONS**

On the enlargement of the capillary in the top right figure:

1. Color the endothelial cells of the capillary Ⓐ.
2. Use a light color (such as yellow) to color the interstitial fluid Ⓘ.
3. Lightly shade the red blood cells Ⓗ and the tissue cells Ⓙ.
4. Use bright, contrasting colors for oxygen Ⓖ and carbon dioxide Ⓚ.

✐ **COLORING INSTRUCTIONS**

On the bottom figure:

1. Color one diagram before moving to the next.
2. Color the walls of the vein Ⓛ, skeletal muscle Ⓜ, the valves Ⓝ, and the arrows representing blood flow Ⓞ.

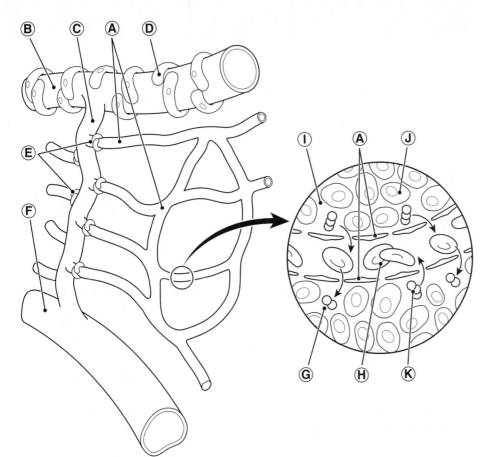

A. capillary bed
B. arteriole
C. metarteriole
D. smooth muscle
E. precapillary
   sphincter
F. venule
G. oxygen
H. red blood cell
I. interstitial fluid
J. tissue cell
K. carbon dioxide
L. vein
M. skeletal muscle
N. valves
O. blood flow

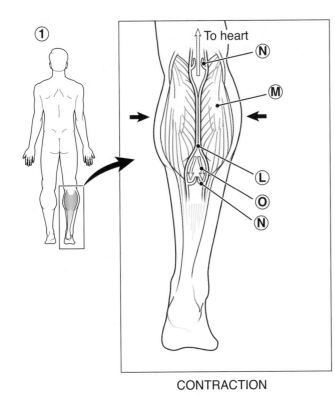

CONTRACTION

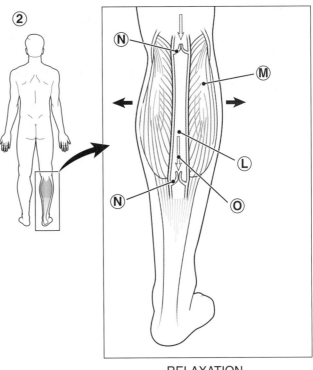

RELAXATION

CHAPTER 9

The Lymphatic System and Immunity

Coloring Exercise 9-1 ➤ **The Lymphatic and Cardiovascular Systems**

Functions of the Lymphatic System

- Fluid balance
  - Net fluid loss from capillaries into interstitial fluid
  - Lymph system returns excess fluid from tissues to the circulation
- Protection
  - Lymph passes through lymph nodes, containing many immune cells
  - Lymphatic system protects against pathogens and often destroys traveling cancerous cells
- Fat absorption
  - Dietary fat from the digestive system is absorbed into lymphatic capillaries

Flow of Blood and Lymph

1. Deoxygenated blood flows from the **right heart** (A), through **pulmonary arteries/arterioles** (B) into **pulmonary capillaries** (C). Oxygenated blood flows from the **left heart** (D) through **systemic arteries/arterioles** (E) into **systemic capillaries** (F).

2. Water and dissolved substances leave the capillaries into the interstitial fluid.

3. Interstitial fluid (now called **lymph** (G)) enters blind-ended **lymphatic capillaries** (H).

4. Lymph passes through one or more **lymphatic vessels** (I) and **lymph nodes** (J). Lymphatic vessels contain **valves** (K) to ensure flow towards the heart, not away from it.

5. All lymph is returned to the **systemic venous circulation** (L) (not the **pulmonary veins** (M)).

✎ COLORING INSTRUCTIONS

Color each part and its name at the same time, using the same color. On the main figure:

1. Color the parts of the circulatory system. Use variants of red for segments carrying oxygenated blood (D), (E), (M), variants of blue for segments carrying deoxygenated blood (A), (B), (L), and variants of purple for the capillary beds (C), (F).

2. Use a dark color for the arrows representing lymph (G).

3. Follow the lymph as it flows through the lymphatic system (I) to (J). Use a dark color for the valves (K).

On the smaller figure: Color all elements of this magnified view of a systemic capillary bed and the associated lymph vessels.

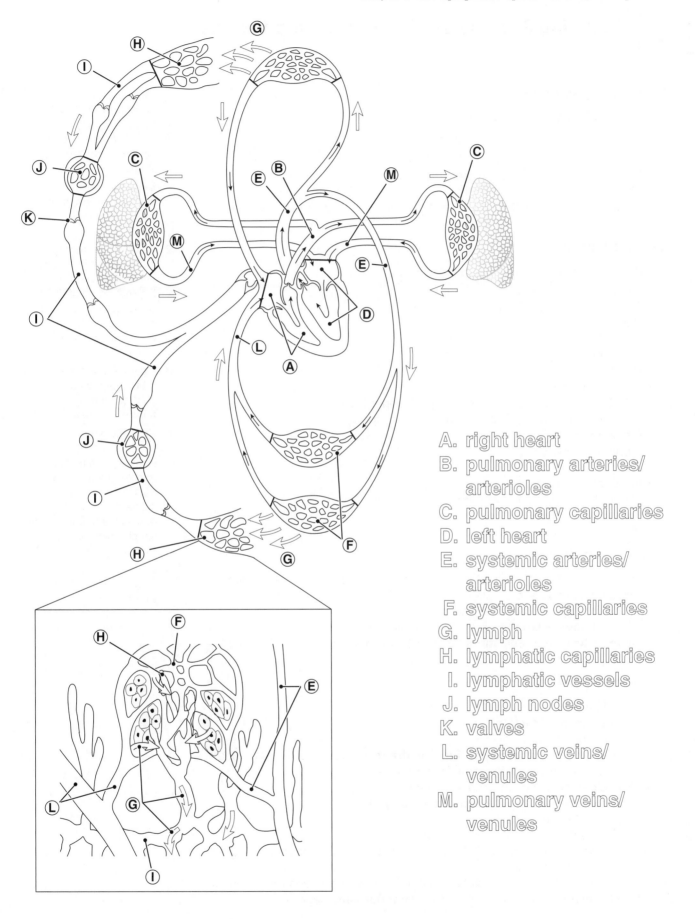

A. right heart
B. pulmonary arteries/
   arterioles
C. pulmonary capillaries
D. left heart
E. systemic arteries/
   arterioles
F. systemic capillaries
G. lymph
H. lymphatic capillaries
 I. lymphatic vessels
J. lymph nodes
K. valves
L. systemic veins/
   venules
M. pulmonary veins/
   venules

Coloring Exercise 9-2 ➤ Lymphatic Vessels

Lymphatic Vessels

- Receive lymph from lymphatic capillaries
- Can be superficial (just under skin) or deep
- Named after the region they drain, for example:
  - **Mammary** vessels Ⓐ: drain breast region
  - **Tibial** vessels Ⓑ: drain lower leg
  - **Femoral** vessels Ⓒ: drain thigh (also receive lymph from tibial vessels)

Lymph Nodes

- Lymph passes through multiple lymph nodes
- Nodes named by their location, for instance
  - **Occipital** Ⓓ: back of head
  - **Cervical** Ⓔ: neck region
  - **Parotid** Ⓕ: jaw/cheek
  - **Mandibular** Ⓖ: chin
  - **Cubital** Ⓗ: elbow
  - **Axillary** Ⓘ: armpit
    - Receives lymph from mammary gland, upper limb
    - Sometimes removed along with mammary tumors
  - **Mesenteric** Ⓙ: internal organs
  - **Lumbar** Ⓚ: back
  - **Iliac** Ⓛ: pelvis
  - **Inguinal** Ⓜ: groin area
    - Receive lymph from lower limb
  - **Popliteal** Ⓝ: knee

Lymphatic Trunks

- After the "last" (most proximal) lymph node, lymphatic vessels merge into **lymphatic trunks,** for example
  - Left/right **jugular** trunks Ⓞ: drain head, neck
  - Left/right **subclavian** trunks Ⓟ: drain upper limbs
  - Left/right **bronchomediastinal** trunks Ⓠ: drain thorax

Lymphatic Ducts

- All lymphatic trunks drain into one of two ducts
  - **Right lymphatic duct** Ⓡ
    - Very short (2.5 cm)
    - Receives lymph from **upper right quadrant** Ⓢ, including the right jugular, subclavian, and bronchomediastinal trunks
  - **Thoracic duct** Ⓣ (or left lymphatic duct)
    - Receives lymph from the **rest of the body** Ⓤ
    - Begins at **cisterna chyli** Ⓥ
      - Receives lymph from pelvis, lower limbs
    - Proximal end receives lymph from the left jugular, subclavian, and bronchomediastinal trunks
  - Ducts drain into left or right **subclavian vein** Ⓦ, which drains into the right or left **brachiocephalic** vein Ⓧ and the **superior vena cava** Ⓨ

✍ COLORING INSTRUCTIONS

Color each figure part and its name at the same time, using the same color. Color both figures together.

1. Use dark colors to outline several lymph vessels in each region (Ⓐ to Ⓒ).
2. Color nodes from different regions (Ⓓ to Ⓝ); not all nodes are labeled. Some of the nodes are only labeled on one side—try to color them on both sides.
3. Lightly shade the background of the upper right quadrant Ⓢ and of the rest of the body Ⓤ.
4. Color the lymphatic trunks and ducts (Ⓞ to Ⓡ, Ⓣ). It will be difficult to color the trunks and ducts on the large diagram. You can try to outline the structures, or simply color them on the enlarged view.
5. Color the veins and superior vena cava (Ⓦ to Ⓨ).

Lymph Vessels

A. mammary
B. tibial
C. femoral

Lymph nodes

D. occipital
E. cervical
F. parotid
G. mandibular

H. cubital
I. axillary
J. mesenteric
K. lumbar

L. iliac
M. inguinal
N. popliteal

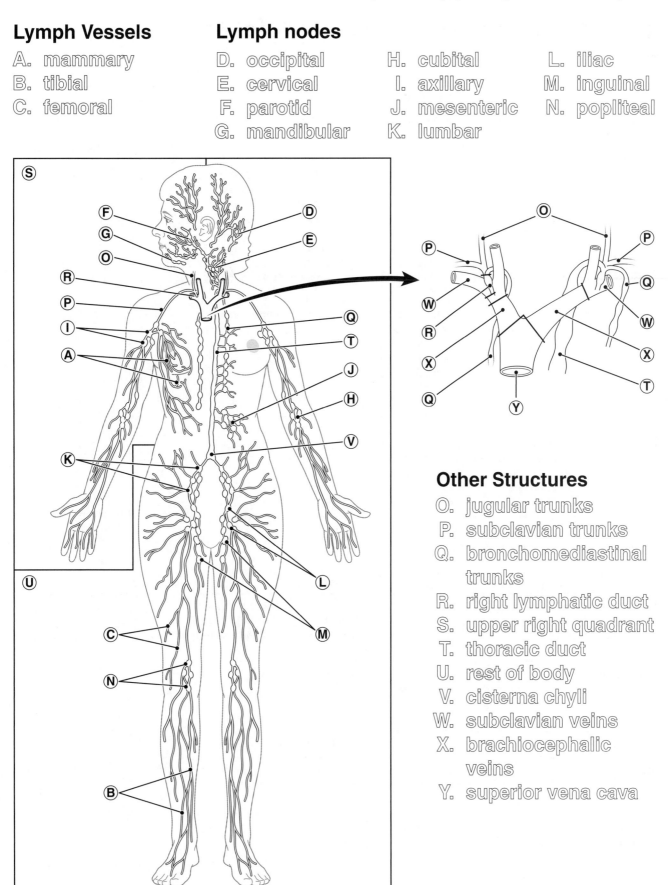

Other Structures

O. jugular trunks
P. subclavian trunks
Q. bronchomediastinal
trunks
R. right lymphatic duct
S. upper right quadrant
T. thoracic duct
U. rest of body
V. cisterna chyli
W. subclavian veins
X. brachiocephalic
veins
Y. superior vena cava

Coloring Exercise 9-3 ➤ Lymphoid Tissues

	Structure	Location	Function
Lymph nodes Ⓐ	See below	See below	Filter lymph
Spleen Ⓑ	Outer capsule of elastic connective tissue and smooth muscle; filled with soft pulp containing phagocytes and lymphocytes	Left hypochondriac region of the abdomen	Destroys worn-out blood cells; serves as blood reservoir; produces blood cells before birth; resident phagocytes cleanse blood of cell debris and impurities
Thymus Ⓒ	Gland; atrophies in adults	Superior thorax, under the sternum	Matures T lymphocytes
Tonsils	Tissue masses in the pharynx; deep grooves trap pathogens	**Palatine** Ⓓ**:** soft palate; **pharyngeal** Ⓔ (adenoids): behind the nose; **lingual** Ⓕ**:** back of tongue	Attack pathogens that are inhaled or swallowed
Appendix Ⓖ	Fingerlike tube	Attached to large intestine	Helps maintain gastro-intestinal microbes
Mucosal-associated lymphoid tissue (MALT)	Lymphoid tissue masses associated with mucous membranes	Linings of digestive, respiratory tracts; **Peyer patches** Ⓗ found in small intestine	Counteract infectious agents

Anatomy of a Lymph Node

	Structure	Function
Lymphatic vessels Ⓘ Ⓙ	Thin-walled vessels; contain valves	Convey lymph in (**afferent** Ⓘ) and out (**efferent** Ⓙ) of lymph node; **valves** Ⓚ ensure one-way **lymph flow** Ⓛ
Capsule Ⓜ	Connective tissue; extensions into the node are **trabeculae** Ⓝ; indented portion is the **hilum** Ⓞ	Supports lymph node
Sinuses Ⓟ	Channels	Permit lymph flow through node
Medullary cords Ⓠ	Colonies of B-cells, macrophages; no germinal centers	Filter lymph of impurities (pathogens, cancer cells)
Cortical nodules Ⓡ	Aggregates of B cells; contain **germinal centers** Ⓢ	B cells proliferate in germinal centers

✍ **COLORING INSTRUCTIONS**

Color each figure part and its name at the same time, using the same color. On the top figure: Color each lymphoid organ. The figure shows many lymph nodes; color a few of them.

✍ **COLORING INSTRUCTIONS**

On the bottom figure:

1. Color the arrows representing lymph flow Ⓛ.

2. Color the capsule Ⓜ in cross section and surrounding the node. Color the circle that indicates the location of the hilum Ⓞ, and color the trabeculae Ⓝ.

3. Color the lymphatic vessels (Ⓘ and Ⓙ). Note that there are more afferent vessels than efferent vessels. Use a dark color for the valves Ⓚ.

4. Color the germinal centers (Ⓢ; try to find all 6). Color the medullary cords Ⓠ and cortical nodules Ⓡ. You can distinguish them by the presence of germinal centers.

5. Color the sinuses Ⓟ.

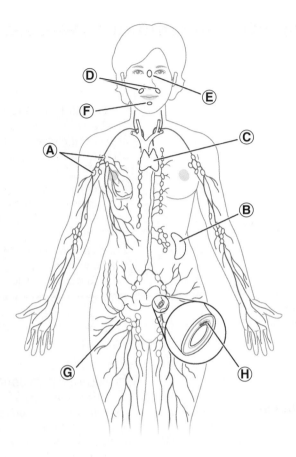

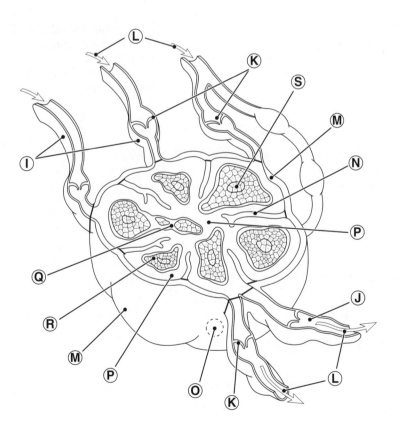

A. lymph nodes
B. spleen
C. thymus
D. palatine tonsils
E. pharyngeal tonsil
F. lingual tonsil
G. appendix
H. Peyer patches
 I. afferent vessel
 J. efferent vessel
K. valves
L. lymph flow
M. capsule
N. trabeculae
O. hilum
P. sinuses
Q. medullary cords
R. cortical nodules
S. germinal centers

Nonspecific and Immune Defenses

- Immune defenses: defends against specific targets
  - Uses lymphocytes (see Coloring Exercises 9-5 to 9-7)
- Nonspecific defenses: defend against any target

Nonspecific Defenses

- Physical defenses
  - Barriers (e.g., **skin** (A)) stop **pathogens** (B) from entering body
  - Mucus traps irritants and microbes
- Chemical defenses
  - Secretions (e.g., **sweat** (C)) wash away pathogens
  - Secretions contain enzymes, other chemicals
  - **Complement** (D): 20 blood proteins; when activated they
    - poke holes in pathogen cell membranes, destroying cell
    - enhance phagocytosis
    - promote **inflammation** (E)
    - attract **macrophages** (F)
- Cellular defenses
  - **Macrophages** (F) (derived from monocytes) and **neutrophils** (G) remove foreign material by phagocytosis
  - **Natural killer (NK) cells** (H) (lymphocyte-like cell) recognize cancer cells and **virus-infected** cells (I)
    - Kills cells by disrupting their plasma membrane

Site	Actions
Eyes (J)	• Tears contain antibiotic chemicals, wash away contaminants
Lymph nodes (K)	• Contain many macrophages, natural killer cells • Natural killer cells attack cancer cells, virus-infected cells
Skin (A)	• Physical barrier
Respiratory tract (L)	• Mucus entraps foreign material • Epithelial cell cilia transport contaminated mucus to throat • Coughing expels contaminated mucus • Macrophages in alveoli phagocytose invaders
Blood (M)	• Contains neutrophils, monocytes (macrophage precursors) • Contains complement proteins
Bone marrow (N)	• Site of white blood cell production
Liver (O)	• Contains many macrophages (Kupffer cells)
Spleen (P)	• Contains many macrophages, NK cells
Digestive tract (Q)	• Gastric acid, bile, and enzymes destroy pathogens • Normal flora (bacteria) compete with invading bacteria for nutrients
Urogenital tract (R)	• Acidic urine and reproductive tract secretions inactivate and wash away pathogens

✍ **COLORING INSTRUCTIONS**

Color each figure part and its name at the same time, using the same color. On the top left figure:

1. Color the microbes (B) that penetrated the natural barriers of skin (A) and sweat (C).

2. Use red to indicate the inflammation (E) surrounding the injury.

3. Color the nonimmune defenses mobilized to attack the pathogen (D), (F), (G).

✍ **COLORING INSTRUCTIONS**

On the top right figure, color the virus-infected cell (I) and the natural killer cell (H) that is breaking down the infected cell's membrane.

✍ **COLORING INSTRUCTIONS**

On the bottom figure, color the different organs involved in non specific immune defenses.

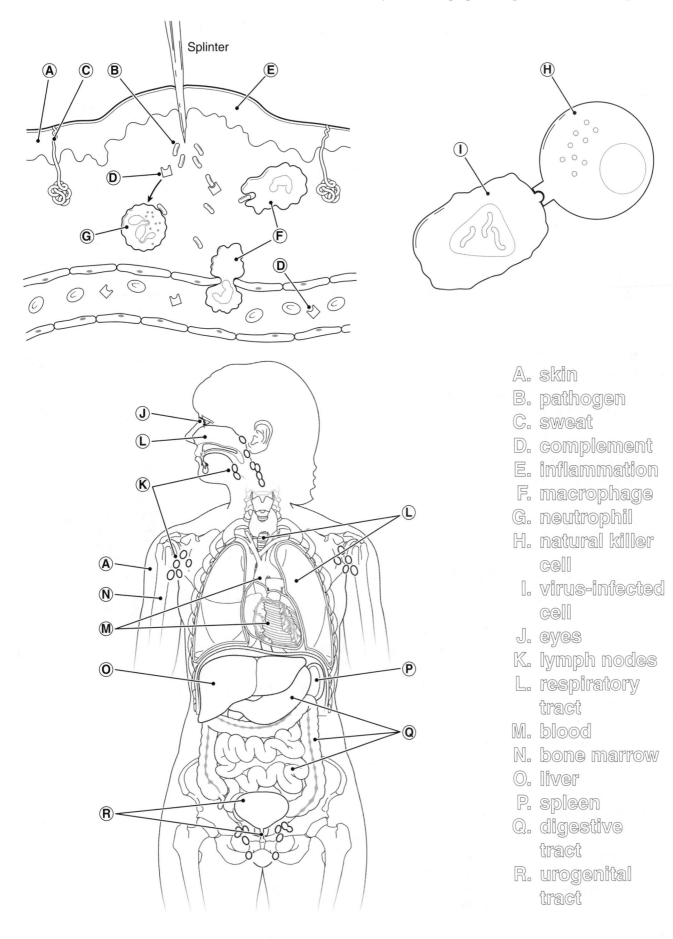

A. skin
B. pathogen
C. sweat
D. complement
E. inflammation
F. macrophage
G. neutrophil
H. natural killer cell
I. virus-infected cell
J. eyes
K. lymph nodes
L. respiratory tract
M. blood
N. bone marrow
O. liver
P. spleen
Q. digestive tract
R. urogenital tract

Coloring Exercise 9-5 ➤ Immunity: Antigens and the Cellular Response

Specific Immunity and Antigens

- **Antigen** Ⓐ: molecule that induces an immune reaction
  - Self antigens: normally found in the body
  - Foreign antigens: not normally found in the body
- Immune responses are directed against a specific foreign antigen

MHC Proteins

- Special self antigens expressed in cell membranes; associated with foreign antigens from internalized pathogens
- **MHC I** Ⓑ: all cells
  - MHC I + foreign antigen signals that cell is infected and must be destroyed
- **MHC II** Ⓒ: **antigen-presenting cells** Ⓓ (see below)
  - MHC II + foreign antigen signals other cells to attack antigen

Lymphocytes and Immunity

- **Immature lymphocytes** Ⓔ mature into B or T cells
- **B cells** Ⓕ: mature in **bone marrow** Ⓖ
  - Secrete **antibodies** Ⓗ (humoral immunity: Coloring Exercise 9-6)
- T cells: mature in **thymus** Ⓘ
  - **Helper T cells** Ⓙ: promote immune responses
  - **Cytotoxic T cells** Ⓚ: cell-mediated immunity (below)
  - **Regulatory T cells** Ⓛ: suppress immune responses
- B cells and T cells exist to bind EVERY possible antigen
- B cells and T cells that recognize self antigens are usually destroyed before they are released into the blood

Helper T Cells and Antigen Presentation

Macrophages "present" antigens to helper T cells to induce an immune reaction against the antigen

1. **Macrophages** Ⓓ ingest **pathogen** Ⓜ into vesicle
2. Vesicle fuses with **lysosome** Ⓝ, forming a **phagocytic vesicle** Ⓞ; lysosomal enzymes digest pathogen into **antigens** Ⓐ
3. Antigens bound to MHC proteins Ⓒ are expressed on the macrophage membrane
4. **T cell receptor** Ⓟ binds antigen/MHC II complex
5. T cell is **activated** Ⓠ, and begins to secrete interleukins
   - **Interleukins** Ⓡ stimulate B cell Ⓕ, T cell Ⓚ (step 6, below), and macrophage Ⓓ activity

Cell-Mediated Immunity

6. Cytotoxic T cells kill virus-infected or cancerous cells
   a. **Infected cells** Ⓢ express **MHC I** Ⓑ proteins on their surface, bound to the foreign **antigen** Ⓐ (viral or cancerous)
   b. **T cell receptor** Ⓟ binds antigen-MHCI complex; cytotoxic T cell pokes holes in infected **cell membrane** Ⓣ, causing cell lysis and death

✎ **COLORING INSTRUCTIONS**
Color each figure part and its name at the same time, using the same color. On the top figure:

1. Lightly shade the bone marrow Ⓖ. Color the immature lymphocytes Ⓔ and the B cells Ⓕ. Use a dark color to outline the antibodies Ⓗ produced by B cells.
2. Color the thymus Ⓘ. Color the three types of T cells (Ⓙ to Ⓛ).

✎ **COLORING INSTRUCTIONS**
On the bottom figure:

1. Color all the elements of each drawing as you go through steps 1–6 in the narrative. Note that not all of the elements are labeled in every drawing.
2. Use closely related colors for the pathogen Ⓜ and the antigen Ⓐ, for the lysosome Ⓝ and the phagocytic vesicle Ⓞ and for the helper T cell Ⓙ and the activated helper T cell Ⓠ.

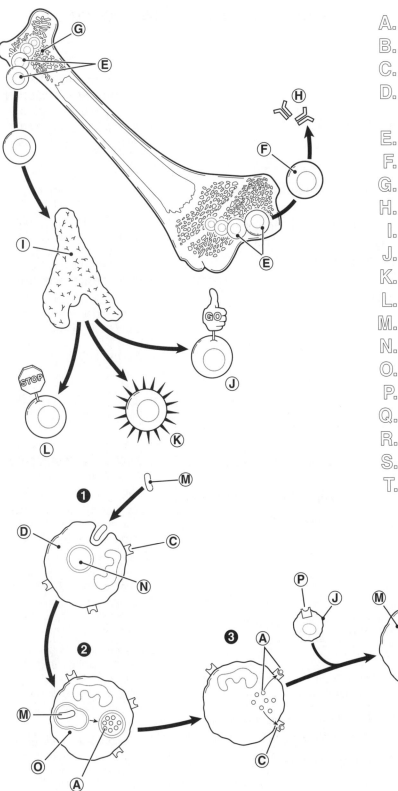

A. antigen
B. MHC I
C. MHC II
D. antigen-presenting
   cell (macrophage)
E. immature lymphocyte
F. B cells
G. bone marrow
H. antibodies
I. thymus
J. helper T cell
K. cytotoxic T cell
L. regulatory T cell
M. pathogen
N. lysosome
O. phagocytic vesicle
P. T cell receptor
Q. activated helper T cell
R. interleukin
S. infected cell
T. dissolving cell membrane

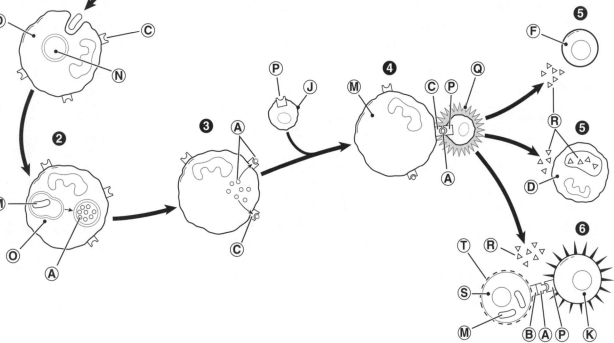

Coloring Exercise 9-6 ➤ Immunity: Humoral Response

Humoral Immunity

- Mediated by B-lymphocytes
- Uses antibodies to attack bacteria (especially) and viruses

B-Lymphocyte Activation

1. **B cell** Ⓐ encounters "its" **antigen** Ⓑ; antigen binds **membrane receptors** Ⓒ and B-cell is activated
2. **Activated B-cell** Ⓐ1 proliferates into many identical B-cells (**clones** Ⓐ2)
3. Some clones differentiate into **plasma cells** Ⓐ3
   - Produce and secrete **antibodies** Ⓓ into bloodstream
   - Short life-span
4. Some clones differentiate into **memory cells** Ⓐ4
   - Do not produce antibodies
   - Long life span
   - Can rapidly differentiate into plasma cells the next time the antigen is encountered

Antibody Actions

- **Prevention of attachment** Ⓔ: antibodies block **viruses** Ⓕ from attaching to body cells
- **Clumping** Ⓖ: a clump formed by **bacteria** Ⓗ and antibodies is easily recognized and ingested by **macrophages** Ⓘ
- **Neutralization** Ⓙ: antibodies prevent **bacterial toxins** Ⓚ from harming cells
- Enhance **phagocytosis** Ⓛ: antibodies help macrophages attach to invader
- Antibodies activate **complement** Ⓜ to destroy cell
- Antibodies activate **natural killer cells** Ⓝ to destroy cell

Antibody Types

Class	Location	Function
IgG	Most abundant type in plasma	Ⓙ, Ⓛ, Ⓜ
IgA	Saliva, tears, breast milk, sweat, mucus	Ⓔ: Prevents pathogens from attaching to mucous membranes
IgM	Blood and lymph; B cell membrane	Ⓖ and Ⓜ: First responder to infection; may be B-cell antigen membrane receptor
IgD	B cell membrane	May be B cell membrane antigen receptor
IgE	Mast cell membranes, secreted by some plasma cells	Involved in inflammation, allergy parasitic infestations

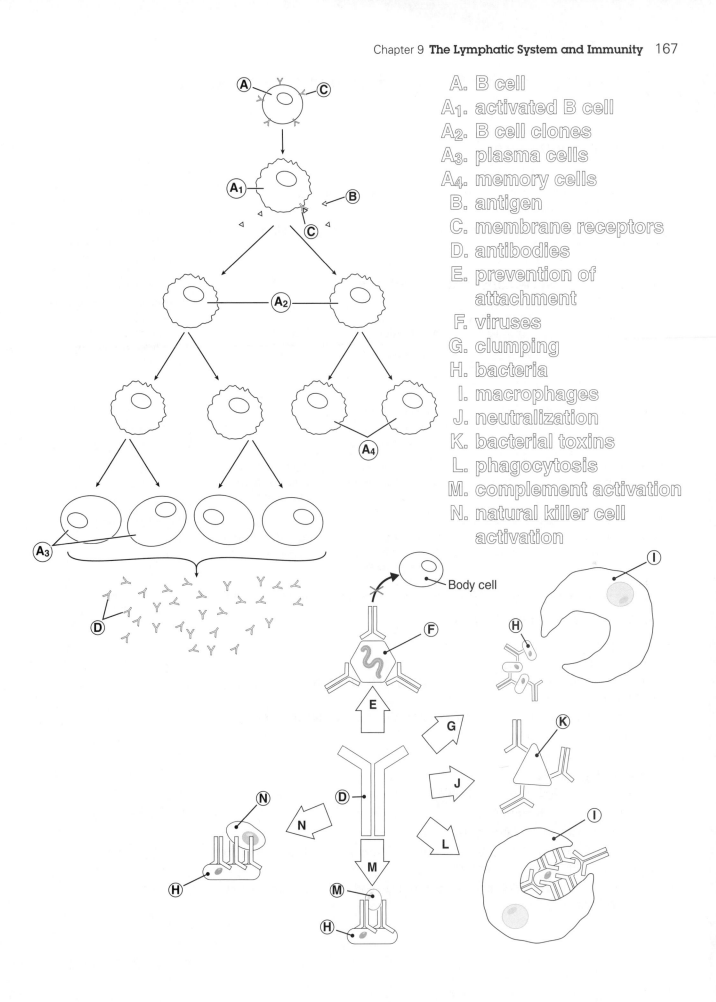

A. B cell
A₁. activated B cell
A₂. B cell clones
A₃. plasma cells
A₄. memory cells
B. antigen
C. membrane receptors
D. antibodies
E. prevention of
   attachment
F. viruses
G. clumping
H. bacteria
 I. macrophages
J. neutralization
K. bacterial toxins
L. phagocytosis
M. complement activation
N. natural killer cell
   activation

Body cell

Coloring Exercise 9-7 ➤ Hypersensitivity Diseases

Hypersensitivity Diseases

- Exaggerated immune responses
- Allergy: immune response to environmental substance that is usually harmless (e.g., pollen, certain foods)
- Autoimmune disease: immune response to self antigens (e.g., multiple sclerosis, type I diabetes mellitus)

Mechanisms of Hypersensitivity Reactions

	Name	Lymphocyte Involved	Mechanism	Examples
Type I	Immediate hypersensitivity	B cells	See below	Hay fever
Type II	Cytotoxic hypersensitivity	B cells	Antibodies attach directly to body cells; inflammation or cell destruction	Myasthenia gravis
Type III	Immune complex hypersensitivity	B cells	Antigen-antibody complex activates complement, inflammation	Most autoimmune diseases, allergic pneumonia
Type IV	Cellular (delayed) hypersensitivity	Cytotoxic T cells	T cells attack self antigens that are similar to foreign antigens	Contact dermatitis (poison ivy)

Immediate Hypersensitivity Response

Example: hay fever

First Exposure

1. Normally harmless **antigen** Ⓐ (called an allergen) binds **receptor** Ⓑ on **B lymphocyte** Ⓒ
2. B lymphocyte is activated (Coloring Exercise 9-6); produces **plasma cells** Ⓓ
3. Plasma cells produce **IgE** Ⓔ
4. IgE binds **mast cells** Ⓕ

Subsequent Exposures

5. **Antigen** Ⓐ binds **IgE** Ⓔ on **mast cells** Ⓕ
6. Mast cells release **histamine** Ⓖ
7. Histamine irritates **nerve endings** Ⓗ (itching)
8. Histamine causes **blood vessels** Ⓘ to **dilate** Ⓙ and become leaky (swelling, redness, possibly low blood pressure)
9. Histamine causes **bronchioles** Ⓚ to **constrict** Ⓛ and produce more **mucus** Ⓜ (wheezing, coughing)

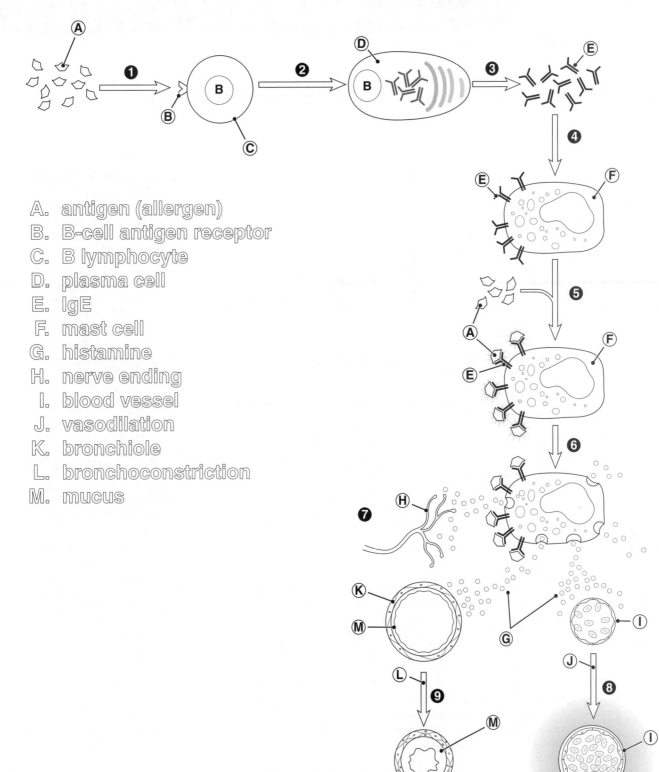

A. antigen (allergen)
B. B-cell antigen receptor
C. B lymphocyte
D. plasma cell
E. IgE
F. mast cell
G. histamine
H. nerve ending
 I. blood vessel
J. vasodilation
K. bronchiole
L. bronchoconstriction
M. mucus

CHAPTER 10

The Respiratory System

Coloring Exercise 10-1 ➤ The Respiratory System

Functions

- Brings oxygen into the body to fuel working cells
- Expels carbon dioxide produced by working cells
- Regulates acid-base balance

Components of the Respiratory System

Component	Structure	Function
Nasal cavity Ⓐ	Mucous membrane-lined cavities	Warm and moisten air; traps foreign bodies in hairs and mucus; sense of smell
Sinuses Ⓑ, Ⓒ	Air-filled spaces in bone	Lighten skull
Pharynx	Muscular tube divided into **nasopharynx** Ⓓ, **oropharynx** Ⓔ, **laryngeal pharynx** Ⓕ	Transports air into trachea and food/liquids into **esophagus** Ⓙ
Epiglottis Ⓖ	Leaf-shaped cartilage	Covers larynx during swallowing; prevents food entry into lungs
Larynx Ⓗ	Cartilaginous structure	Contains vocal cords for speech; joins pharynx and trachea
Trachea Ⓘ	Cartilage-reinforced muscular tube	Transports air to bronchi
Bronchi Ⓚ	Trachea divides into two bronchi (which subdivide) serving the **right** Ⓛ and **left** Ⓜ **lungs**	Transport air to bronchioles
Bronchioles Ⓝ	Smallest branches of the bronchi; walls contain smooth muscle	Transport air to alveoli
Diaphragm Ⓞ	Strong muscle	Changes thoracic volume to enable breathing
Pleura	Connective tissue double membrane; **visceral pleura** Ⓟ attached to lung; **parietal pleura** Ⓠ attached to **chest wall** Ⓡ; fluid-filled **pleural space** Ⓢ separates two layers	Pleural membranes slide over each other, enabling the lungs to expand and contract as thoracic volume changes
Alveoli Ⓣ	Clustered, interlinked air sacs (see below)	Sites of gas exchange

Alveoli

- Air sac wall consists of a single layer of squamous epithelium
  - **Type I pneumocytes** Ⓤ: flat cells, sites of gas exchange
  - **Type II pneumocytes** Ⓥ: secrete surfactant (makes lungs easier to inflate)
- Many **capillaries** Ⓦ between air sacs

COLORING INSTRUCTIONS

Read all the instructions before beginning. Color each structure and its name at the same time, using the same color.

1. Color the components of the respiratory system (and associated structures) as you go through the table.

2. If you like, lightly shade the table row with the same color used for the structure.

3. Use related colors for the two sinuses (Ⓑ and Ⓒ) and the three parts of the pharynx (Ⓓ to Ⓕ).

3. Do not color the lungs (Ⓛ and Ⓜ) in the large diagram, but color them in the cross-section of the thorax.

4. Use dark colors to outline the pleural membranes (Ⓟ and Ⓠ) and a contrasting color for the pleural space (Ⓢ).

A. nasal cavity
B. frontal sinus
C. sphenoidal sinus
D. nasopharynx
E. oropharynx
F. laryngeal pharynx
G. epiglottis
H. larynx
I. trachea
J. esophagus
K. bronchi
L. right lung
M. left lung
N. bronchioles
O. diaphragm
P. visceral pleura
Q. parietal pleura
R. chest wall
S. pleural space
T. alveoli
U. type I pneumocyte
V. type II pneumocyte
W. capillary

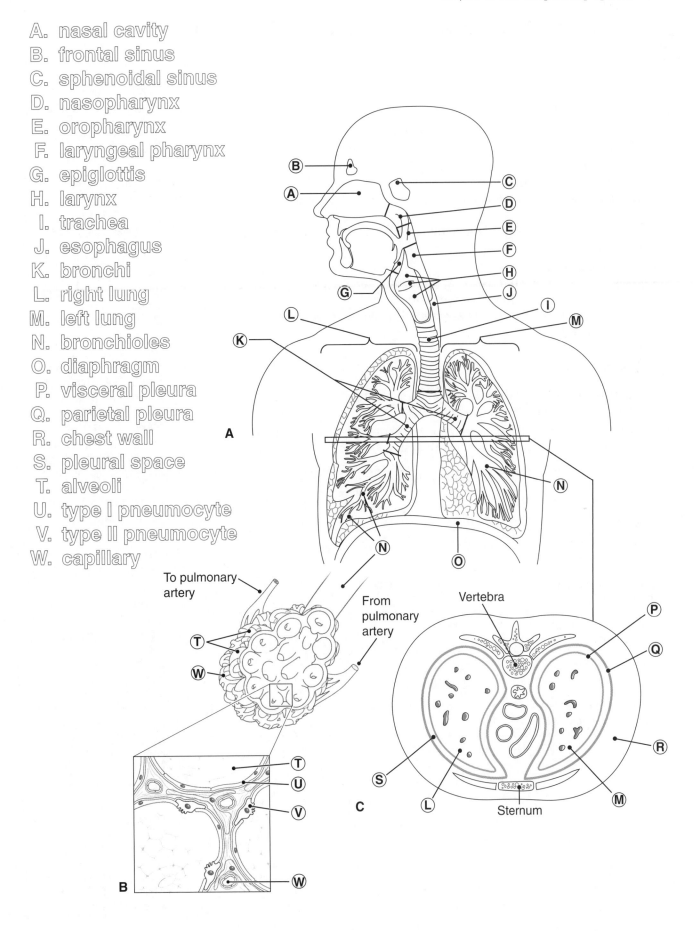

To pulmonary artery

From pulmonary artery

Vertebra

Sternum

A

B

C

Coloring Exercise 10-2 ➤ Phases of Respiration

Phases of Respiration

- **Pulmonary Ventilation** Ⓐ
  - Moves air in and out of the alveoli of the **lungs** Ⓑ
  - **Inhaled air** Ⓒ is high in oxygen, low in carbon dioxide
  - **Exhaled air** Ⓓ is low in oxygen, high in carbon dioxide
- **External Gas Exchange** Ⓔ
  - **Oxygen** Ⓕ and **carbon dioxide** Ⓖ move between the **lungs** Ⓑ and the blood
  - Blood arriving in the lungs is **deoxygenated** Ⓗ, blood leaving the lungs is **oxygenated** Ⓘ
- **Internal Gas Exchange** Ⓙ
  - **Oxygen** Ⓕ and **carbon dioxide** Ⓖ move between the blood and the cells of the **upper body** Ⓚ and the **lower body** Ⓛ
  - Blood arriving in the tissues is **oxygenated** Ⓘ, blood leaving the tissues is **deoxygenated** Ⓗ

Diffusion of Gases

- Gases (**oxygen** Ⓕ and **carbon dioxide** Ⓖ) can diffuse through the thin, epithelial walls of **alveoli** Ⓑ1 and **capillaries** Ⓜ1.
- Diffusion occurs down the concentration gradient (from the area of higher concentration to the area of lower concentration)

	Lungs/Alveoli	Tissues
Oxygen concentration in arriving blood	Low	High
Alveolar/Tissue oxygen concentration	High	Low
Oxygen gradient/direction of movement Ⓕ	From lungs to blood	From blood to tissues
Carbon dioxide concentration in arriving blood	High	Low
Alveolar/tissue carbon dioxide concentration	Low	High
Carbon dioxide gradient/ direction of movement Ⓖ	From blood to lungs	From tissues to blood

A. pulmonary ventilation
B. lungs (alveoli)
B₁. alveolar wall
C. inhaled air
D. exhaled air
E. external gas exchange

F. oxygen
G. carbon dioxide
H. deoxygenated blood
I. oxygenated blood
J. internal gas exchange
K. upper body cells

L. lower body cells
M. capillary
M₁. capillary wall

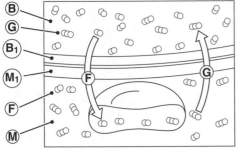

Coloring Exercise 10-3 ➤ Ventilation

Ventilation

- Movement of air in and out of the **lungs** Ⓐ
- Air moves down pressure gradients created by volume changes in the lungs
  - Increased lung volume Ⓑ = decreased pressure Ⓒ
  - Decreased lung volume Ⓓ = increased pressure Ⓔ
  - Think of squeezing a tube of toothpaste: squeezing reduces the volume, increasing the pressure (and toothpaste squirts out down the gradient)
- Pleural membranes stick thorax and lungs together, so they change volume together

Inhalation Ⓕ: *The Active Phase*

- Thoracic and **lung volume increase** Ⓑ
- As lungs expand, the **pressure in the lungs decreases** Ⓒ
- Lung pressure drops below atmospheric pressure, creating an inward pressure gradient
- **Air flows into the lungs** Ⓕ down the gradient

Muscle Activity During Inhalation

- **Diaphragm** Ⓖ contracts
  - Abdominal organs pushed downward
- **External intercostal** Ⓗ muscles contract
  - **Rib cage** Ⓘ moves up and out (**sternum** Ⓙ elevates)
- Thorax expands vertically and horizontally
- Stronger contractions = deeper inhalation
  - Accessory muscles of neck and chest can enlarge the thorax even more, resulting in very deep inhalations

Exhalation Ⓚ: *Passive or Active*

- Thorax and lungs recoil back to **smaller volume** Ⓓ
- As lung size decreases, air **pressure in the lungs increases** Ⓔ
- Lung pressure rises above atmospheric pressure, creating a pressure gradient
- **Air flows out of the lungs** Ⓚ down the pressure gradient

Muscle Activity During Relaxed (PASSIVE) Exhalation

- **Diaphragm** Ⓖ relaxes, abdominal organs recoil upward
- **External intercostals** Ⓗ relax
  - **Sternum** Ⓙ moves down
- Thorax volume is reduced

Muscle Activity During Active Exhalation

- **Internal intercostal muscles** Ⓛ contract
  - **Rib cage** Ⓘ moves in and down
- Abdominal muscles contract
  - Abdominal organs pushed upwards against the diaphragm
- Thoracic volume is reduced rapidly and to a greater extent

✎ **COLORING INSTRUCTIONS**

Color each structure and its name at the same time, using the same color. On the top left figure:

1. Lightly shade the lungs Ⓐ.
2. Color the arrows representing airflow Ⓕ and changes in lung volume Ⓑ.
3. Color the symbol representing a change in pressure Ⓒ.

On top right figure:

1. Lightly shade the lungs Ⓐ and the muscles involved in inhalation (Ⓗ and Ⓖ).
2. Color the arrows representing movements of the diaphragm Ⓖ and sternum Ⓙ and the direction of the airflow Ⓕ.
3. Color the lines representing the rib cage Ⓘ before (solid line) and after (dotted line) inhalation.

✎ **COLORING INSTRUCTIONS**

On the bottom left figure:

1. Lightly shade the lungs Ⓐ.
2. Color the arrows representing airflow Ⓚ and changes in lung volume Ⓓ.
3. Color the symbol representing a change in pressure Ⓔ.

On the bottom right figure:

1. Lightly shade the lungs Ⓐ and the muscles involved in exhalation (Ⓛ and Ⓖ). Remember that the diaphragm relaxes during exhalation.
2. Color the arrows representing movements of the diaphragm Ⓖ and the sternum Ⓙ and airflow Ⓚ.
3. Color the lines representing the rib cage Ⓘ before (solid line) and after (dotted line) exhalation.

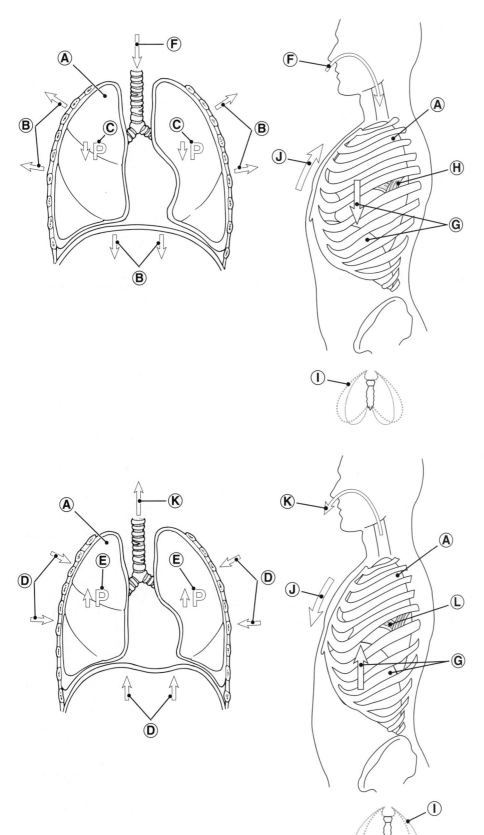

A. lung
B. increased thoracic/lung volume
C. decreased pressure
D. decreased thoracic/lung volume
E. increased pressure
F. inhalation/ inward pressure gradient
G. diaphragm
H. external intercostals
I. rib cage
J. sternum
K. exhalation/ outward pressure gradient
L. internal intercostals

Coloring Exercise 10-4 ➤ Gas Transport

Oxygen Transport

- In the blood, 98% of **oxygen** Ⓐ is carried on the **hemoglobin** molecule Ⓑ, 2% dissolved in plasma
  - Each hemoglobin has four subunits and can carry four oxygen molecules
  - Each red blood cell contains many hemoglobin molecules
  - Oxygen binds hemoglobin when oxygen is abundant (lungs) and dissociates when oxygen is lacking (tissue)
- External gas exchange
  - Oxygen diffuses quickly through epithelial cells Ⓒ of alveoli and capillaries
  - **Oxygen** Ⓐ moves down its **gradient** Ⓓ from the **alveolus** Ⓔ into the **pulmonary capillary** Ⓕ
  - Dissolved oxygen in plasma moves into the **red blood cell** Ⓖ and binds **hemoglobin** Ⓑ
- Internal gas exchange
  - In **tissue capillaries** Ⓗ, oxygen dissociates from **hemoglobin** Ⓑ and moves down its **gradient** Ⓓ into **body cells** Ⓘ

Carbon Dioxide Transport

- In the blood
  - 15% carried on proteins (such as hemoglobin, not shown)
  - 10% dissolved in plasma
  - 75% is carried as **bicarbonate** Ⓚ
    - Carbon dioxide is converted into bicarbonate when carbon dioxide is abundant (tissues)
    - Bicarbonate is converted into carbon dioxide when carbon dioxide is less abundant (lungs)
    - Chemical reaction occurs in red blood cells
- Internal gas exchange
  - **Carbon dioxide** Ⓙ moves down its **gradient** Ⓛ from cells into the **tissue capillary** Ⓗ
  - Most carbon dioxide is combined with **water** Ⓜ to form **carbonic acid** Ⓝ
  - Carbonic acid breaks down into **hydrogen ion** Ⓞ and **bicarbonate** Ⓚ
  - Blood becomes more acidic (more hydrogen ions)
- External gas exchange
  - **Bicarbonate** Ⓚ and **hydrogen ions** Ⓞ are converted back into **carbon dioxide** Ⓙ and **water** Ⓜ
  - **Carbon dioxide** Ⓙ moves down its **gradient** Ⓛ from **pulmonary capillary** Ⓕ to the **alveolus** Ⓔ
  - Blood becomes less acidic (fewer hydrogen ions)

COLORING INSTRUCTIONS

Color each figure part and its name at the same time, using the same color. On the left-hand figures:

1. Color all the elements except oxygen (Ⓐ) of the top diagram, illustrating external gas exchange of oxygen. Note that hemoglobin Ⓑ is represented by a box, and the pulmonary capillaries Ⓕ are shown on the alveolus and in the magnified view. Do not color the epithelial cells Ⓒ. The oxygen gradient is represented by arrow Ⓓ.

2. Follow the oxygen molecules Ⓐ out of the alveolus, into blood cells, and bind to hemoglobin. Then, follow them detaching from the hemoglobin to enter body cells in the bottom figure.

COLORING INSTRUCTIONS

On the right-hand figures:

1. Color all of the elements of the top figure, illustrating internal gas exchange of carbon dioxide. Move from right to left as you color the components of the chemical reaction (Ⓙ, Ⓚ, Ⓜ to Ⓞ). Make sure that you color all of the carbon dioxide molecules, represented by abbreviations or 3 small balls.

2. Color all of the elements of the bottom right-hand figure illustrating external gas exchange of carbon dioxide. Color the components of the chemical reaction from left to right.

A. oxygen
B. hemoglobin
C. epithelial cells
D. oxygen gradient
E. alveolus
F. pulmonary capillary
G. red blood cell
H. tissue capillary

I. body cells
J. carbon dioxide
K. bicarbonate
L. carbon dioxide
   gradient
M. water
N. carbonic acid
O. hydrogen ion

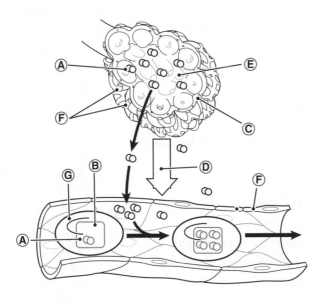

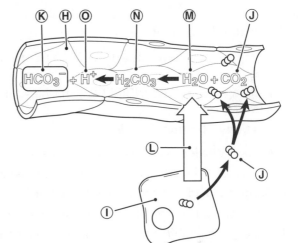

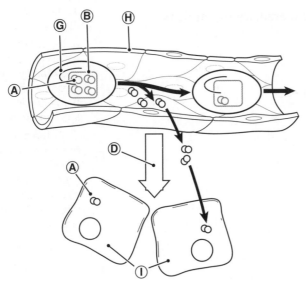

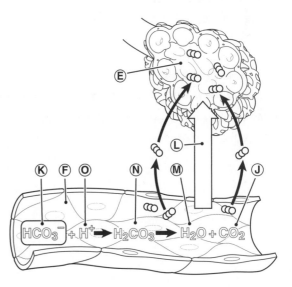

Coloring Exercise 10-5 ➤ Control of Breathing

Nervous Control

- **Medullary rhythmicity area** (A)
  - Controls the muscles of inspiration and expiration
  - Neuron cell bodies located in the **medulla oblongata** (B); axons synapse with spinal nerve cell bodies in the **spinal cord** (C)
  - **Phrenic nerve** (D) sends impulses to the **diaphragm** (E)
  - **Intercostal nerves** (F) send impulses to the **intercostal muscles** (G)
- Respiratory centers in the **pons** (H)
  - Modify the activity of the medullary rhythmicity area
  - **Pneumotaxic center** (I): controls inhalation to prevent lung damage
  - **Apneustic center** (J): promotes longer inhalations

Chemical Control

- Increased **carbon dioxide** (K) is the main stimulus for increased breathing rate
- Carbon dioxide levels INDIRECTLY measured by special neurons (**chemoreceptors** (L))

Detection of Carbon Dioxide

- **Carbon dioxide** (K) levels increase in **cerebral capillaries** (M)
- Carbon dioxide **diffuses** (N) into the **cerebrospinal fluid** (O)
- **Carbon dioxide** (K) combines with **water** (P) to produce **carbonic acid** (Q)
- Carbonic acid breaks down into **bicarbonate** (R) and **hydrogen** (S) ions
- Hydrogen ions **diffuse** (N) into the **medulla oblongata** (B) and activate **chemoreceptor neurons** (L)
- Chemoreceptor neurons activate neurons in the **medullary rhythmicity area** (A)
- Breathing rate increases
- Carbon dioxide levels drop

Oxygen Levels and Breathing Rate (not illustrated)

- **Very** low oxygen levels increase breathing rate
- Only relevant at high altitude and in severe lung disease

COLORING INSTRUCTIONS

Color each figure part and its name at the same time, using the same color. On the top figure:

1. Lightly shade the pons (H), medulla oblongata (B), and spinal cord (C).

2. Use darker colors for the medullary rhythmicity area (A), the spinal nerves ((D) and (F)), and the respiratory muscles ((E) and (G)).

3. Color the pneumotaxic (I) and apneustic (J) centers.

COLORING INSTRUCTIONS

On the bottom figure:

1. Lightly shade the capillary (M), cerebrospinal fluid (O), and medulla oblongata (B).

2. Color the carbon dioxide molecules in the blood (K) and the arrow representing diffusion (N).

3. Color all of the symbols of the chemical reaction converting carbon dioxide (K) and water (P) into carbonic acid (Q), and then into bicarbonate (R) and hydrogen (S).

4. Color the arrow representing hydrogen diffusion (N), the chemoreceptor neurons (L) and the neuron of the medullary rhythmicity area (A).

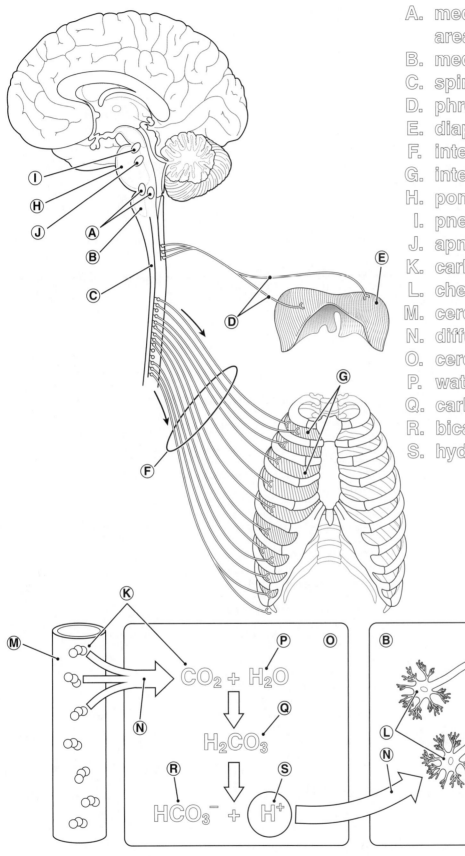

A. medullary rhythmicity area
B. medulla oblongata
C. spinal cord
D. phrenic nerve
E. diaphragm
F. intercostal nerves
G. intercostal muscles
H. pons
I. pneumotaxic center
J. apneustic center
K. carbon dioxide
L. chemoreceptor neurons
M. cerebral capillary
N. diffusion
O. cerebrospinal fluid
P. water
Q. carbonic acid
R. bicarbonate
S. hydrogen

$$CO_2 + H_2O$$
$$H_2CO_3$$
$$HCO_3^- + H^+$$

Coloring Exercise 10-6 ➤ Analysis of Lung Function and Dysfunction

Spirometry

- Measures lung function and helps diagnose lung disease
- Spirometer measures the volume of air exhaled and sometimes inhaled
- Lung volumes are measured directly
- Lung capacities reflect multiple lung volumes

Generation of a Spirograph

- Perform actions that would result in this spirogram reading by:
  - **Quiet breathing** (three breaths) Ⓐ
  - **Deepest possible inhale and exhale** Ⓑ, then two quiet breaths
  - **Deepest possible inhale and normal exhale** Ⓒ, then two quiet breaths
    - At the end of the second normal exhale, **exhale maximally** and let your lungs return to their normal, resting volume Ⓓ
- Forced expiratory volume in 1 second (**FEV1**) Ⓔ: amount of air forcibly exhaled in 1 second

Lung Volumes and Capacities

Name	Average Value	Description
Tidal volume (**TV**) Ⓕ	500 mL (at rest)	Volume of air moving in and out of lungs; increases with exercise
Inspiratory reserve volume (IRV) Ⓖ	2,600 mL	Volume of air forcibly inhaled after normal inhalation
Expiratory reserve volume (ERV) Ⓗ	900 mL	Volume of air forcibly exhaled after a normal exhalation
Residual volume (RV) Ⓘ	1,200 mL	Volume of air remaining in lungs after maximal exhalation (cannot be measured by spirometry)
Vital capacity Ⓙ	4,000 mL	Volume of air forcibly exhaled after maximal inhalation; TV + IRV + ERV
Inspiratory capacity Ⓚ	3,100 mL	IRV + TV
Functional residual capacity Ⓛ	2,100 mL	Volume of air remaining in lungs after normal exhalation; RV + ERV
Total lung capacity Ⓜ	5,200 mL	Total volume of air the lungs can hold; TV + IRV + ERV + RV

Obstructive Lung Disease

- Difficult exhalation due to impaired airflow; reduced **FEV1**

Example: Asthma

- Components of a normal bronchus
  - Small **mucous glands** Ⓝ, **smooth muscle** Ⓞ, and **large lumen** Ⓟ
- Asthma: **inflammation** Ⓠ result in many large **mucous glands** Ⓝ, increased **smooth muscle** Ⓞ
  - **Bronchial lumen** Ⓟ is smaller and obstructed by a **mucus plug** Ⓡ

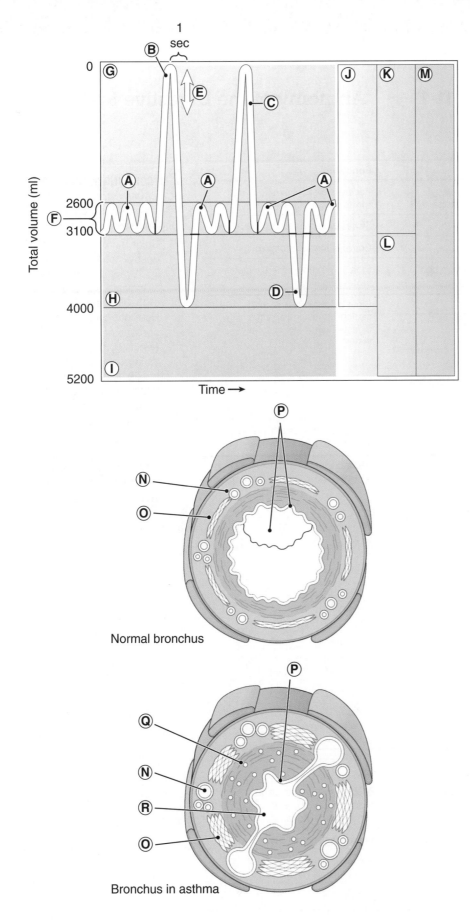

Normal bronchus

Bronchus in asthma

A. quiet breathing
B. deep inhale/ exhale
C. deep inhale/ normal exhale
D. deep exhale
E. FEV1
F. tidal volume
G. inspiratory reserve volume
H. expiratory reserve volume
I. residual volume
J. vital capacity
K. inspiratory capacity
L. functional residual capacity
M. total lung capacity
N. mucous glands
O. smooth muscle
P. lumen
Q. inflammatory cell
R. mucus plug

The Digestive System

Coloring Exercise 11-1 ➤ Anatomy of the Digestive System

Structure	Anatomy	Function
Mouth Ⓐ (Coloring Exercise 11-3)	Includes the tongue, teeth, cheeks, and lips	Receives food; chews food and mixes it with saliva
Pharynx Ⓑ	Muscular tube	Swallows food
Esophagus Ⓒ	Muscular tube	Conveys food to stomach
Stomach Ⓓ (11-4)	J-shaped muscular organ	Stores and churns food; initiates protein digestion
SMALL INTESTINE: (11-6)		Digests fats, proteins, and carbohydrates and absorbs digested nutrients; absorbs water
Duodenum Ⓔ	First 10" of small intestine	
Jejunum Ⓕ	Next 4' of small intestine	
Ileum Ⓖ	Final 6' of small intestine	
Ileocecal valve Ⓗ	Muscular sphincter	Prevents backflow from large intestine to small intestine
LARGE INTESTINE:		Bacteria digest undigested nutrients; absorbs some water
Cecum Ⓘ	Small pouch	
Appendix Ⓙ	Lymphoid tissue	
Ascending colon Ⓚ	Ascends right side towards liver	
Transverse colon Ⓛ	Extends across abdomen	
Descending colon Ⓜ	Descends left side into pelvis	
Sigmoid colon Ⓝ	Projects dorsally in an S-shape	
Tenia coli Ⓞ	Longitudinal muscle	Pulls large intestine into folds
Rectum Ⓟ	Distal portion of large intestine	Temporary storage of food residue
Anus Ⓠ		Expels food residue (feces) from body
Salivary glands	Include the **parotid** Ⓡ, **submandibular** Ⓢ, and **sublingual** Ⓣ **glands**	Saliva moistens food bolus, enables speech, cleanses mouth, and initiates carbohydrate digestion
Pancreas Ⓤ (11-5)	Endocrine/exocrine gland	Produces pancreatic juice
Liver Ⓥ (11-5)	Large reddish brown organ	Produces bile; also has many non-digestive functions
Gallbladder Ⓦ	Muscular sac	Stores bile

✍ **COLORING INSTRUCTIONS**

Color each structure and its name at the same time, using the same color.

1. Color the parts of the digestive tract (Ⓐ through Ⓠ). Draw a small circle to indicate the location of the ileocecal valve Ⓗ. Use light colors for the portions of the large intestine Ⓘ to Ⓝ) and a darker color for the tenia coli Ⓞ. Note that the intestinal segments are separated by lines.

2. Color the accessory organs of digestion (Ⓡ through Ⓦ). Use a dark color for the pancreas Ⓤ, which is behind the stomach.

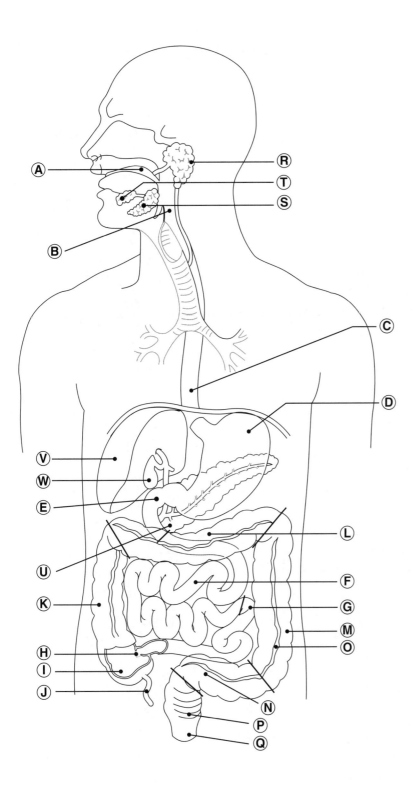

A. mouth
B. pharynx
C. esophagus
D. stomach
E. duodenum
F. jejunum
G. ileum
H. ileocecal valve
 I. cecum
 J. appendix
K. ascending colon
L. transverse colon
M. descending colon
N. sigmoid colon
O. tenia coli
 P. rectum
Q. anus
R. parotid gland
S. submandibular gland
T. sublingual gland
U. pancreas
V. liver
W. gallbladder

Coloring Exercise 11-2 ➤ The Digestive Tract Wall

Components of the Small Intestine Wall

Note that other parts of the digestive tract have similar components

Serosa (A): Outermost Layer
- Serous membrane: squamous epithelium, connective tissue
- Forms part of peritoneum

Muscular Layer
- Smooth (autonomic) muscle
- Outer **circular layer** (B): contracts to constrict lumen
- Inner **longitudinal** (C) layer: contracts to shorten tube
- Contraction controlled by autonomic **nerves** (D) that run between muscle layers
- Stomach (Coloring Exercise 11-4) has an extra muscle layer

Submucosa (E)
- Connective tissue provides structure, support
- **Lymphatic vessels** (F), **blood vessels** (G)
- **Nerves** (D) regulating activity of mucosa
- Mucous glands (not shown)
- **Peyer patches** (H) (lymphatic tissue)

Mucosa (I)
- Contains thin muscular layer (not shown)
- Outer layer of simple columnar cells
  - Some specialized for mucus production (**goblet cells** (J))
  - Most specialized for absorption (**absorptive cells** (K))
  - Some cells secrete hormones (not shown; Coloring Exercise 11-7)
- Surface area for absorption is maximized by
  - Mucosal folds (**plica** (I1))
  - Plica are folded into **villi** (I2)
  - Each absorptive cell has **microvilli** (K1)
- **Submucosa** (E) extends up into each mucosal villus
  - Contains **lymphatic vessel** (F) to absorb fat
  - Contains **blood vessels** (G) to absorb other nutrients
- Mucosa differs between digestive tract organs
  - Mouth/esophagus: squamous epithelial cells, no villi
  - Stomach: columnar cells; mucosa folded into rugae (Coloring Exercise 11-5)
  - Large intestine: columnar cells; no folds

✎ COLORING INSTRUCTIONS

Color each structure and its name at the same time, using the same color.

1. Color the different components of the digestive tract wall on all three diagrams.

2. Use the same color for the terms (I), (I1), and (I2), but only color (I) on the diagrams.

3. Use the same color for the terms (K) and (K1), but only color (K) on the diagrams.

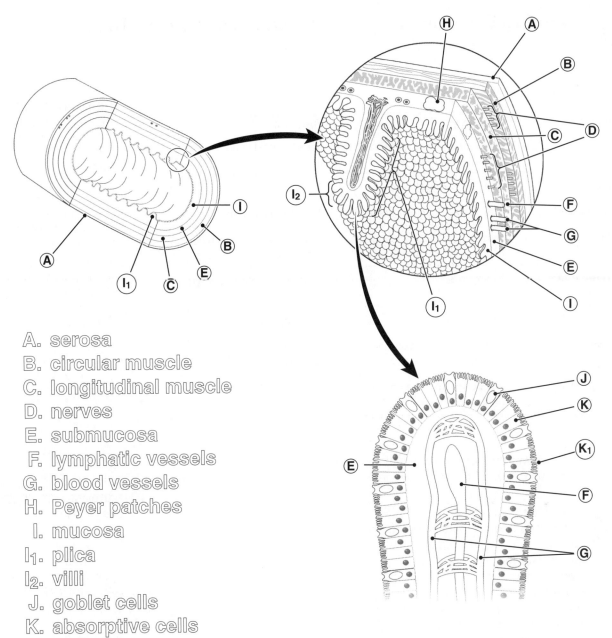

A. serosa
B. circular muscle
C. longitudinal muscle
D. nerves
E. submucosa
F. lymphatic vessels
G. blood vessels
H. Peyer patches
I. mucosa
I$_1$. plica
I$_2$. villi
J. goblet cells
K. absorptive cells
K$_1$. microvilli

Coloring Exercise 11-3 ➤ The Oral Cavity and Teeth

The Mouth

Structure	Anatomy	Function
Upper (A) and **lower** (B) **lips**	Attached to gums; surrounded by orbicularis oris muscle	Speech, mastication (chewing)
Cheeks (C)	Buccinator muscle	Aid in mastication
Hard palate (D)	Maxillae and palatine bones	Aids in mastication
Soft palate (E)	Muscle; contains a V-shaped hanging portion (**uvula** (F))	Soft palate and uvula block nasal cavity during swallowing
Palatopharyngeal arch (G)	Fleshy fold	Joins soft palate to pharynx
Palatine tonsils (H)	Lymphoid tissue	Immune defense
Tongue (I)	Extremely strong skeletal muscle	Manipulates food, taste, swallowing, speech
Gum (gingiva) (J)	Mucous membrane covering tooth sockets	

Teeth

The top figure shows the permanent (adult) dentition (teeth)
- 20 deciduous (baby) teeth appear between 6 months–3 years and fall out by age 12
- In each quadrant, there are:
  - **Central** (K) and **lateral** (L) **incisors**: cut food
  - One **cuspid** (canines) (M): grip and tear food
  - Two **premolars** (bicuspids) (N): grind food
    - replace baby molars
  - Three molars: grind food
    - **First molar** (O1) appears at 6 years of age
    - Molars do not replace any baby teeth
    - **Third molars** (O2); wisdom teeth

Structure of a Molar
- Externally divided into **crown** (P) and **root(s)** (Q)
  - **Periodontal membrane** (a ligament) (R) covers root
  - Teeth anchored in **alveolar bone** (S) of jawbones
    - Bone protected by **gingiva** (J)
- Internal components
  - Outermost layer: **enamel** (T)
    - Covers crown
    - Calcium salts; hardest substance in body
    - Protects tooth from mechanical, chemical stress
  - Middle layer: **dentin** (U)
    - Calcified connective tissue; harder than bone
    - In root region, covered by **cementum** (V)
  - Inner region: **pulp chamber** (W)
    - Connective tissue, blood vessels, nerves
    - **Root canals** (X) are narrow extensions that run down tooth roots

COLORING INSTRUCTIONS
Color each structure and its name at the same time, using the same color. On the top figure:

1. Color parts (A) to (J). Some structures are labeled on only one side; make sure you color them on both sides.
2. Use related colors for the soft palate (E) and the uvula (F).

COLORING INSTRUCTIONS
On the top figure:

1. Color all of the adult teeth. Note that teeth are only labeled in one quadrant. Make sure you color them in all quadrants.
2. Use the same color (or closely related colors) for the molars ((O1) and (O2)).

COLORING INSTRUCTIONS
On the bottom figure:

1. Color the arrows representing the two tooth divisions ((P) and (Q)).
2. Color the internal components of the tooth ((R) to (X)). Use dark colors to outline the periodontal membrane (R), and the cementum (V) that lies just underneath it.

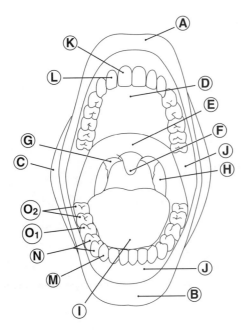

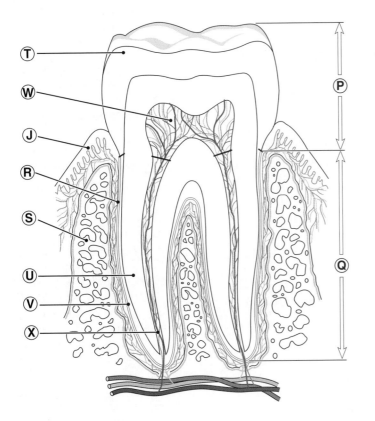

A. upper lip
B. lower lip
C. cheek
D. hard palate
E. soft palate
F. uvula
G. palatopharyngeal arch
H. palatine tonsil
I. tongue
J. gum (gingiva)
K. central incisor
L. lateral incisor
M. cuspid
N. premolars
O_1. first molar
O_2. third molar
P. crown
Q. root
R. preiodontal membrane
S. alveolar bone
T. enamel
U. dentin
V. cementum
W. pulp chamber
X. root canal

Coloring Exercise 11-4 ➤ The Stomach

Anatomy

- Curved, J-shaped organ
  - Inner curve: **lesser curvature** Ⓐ
  - Outer curve: **greater curvature** Ⓑ
- Food enters from the **esophagus** Ⓒ through the **cardiac orifice** Ⓓ
  - Passage controlled by **cardiac** (lower esophageal) **sphincter** Ⓔ
- Food (now mixed into chyme) exits to the **duodenum** Ⓕ through the **pyloric orifice** Ⓖ
  - Passage controlled by **pyloric sphincter** Ⓗ

Three Regions

- Upper **fundus** Ⓘ
  - Above the cardiac sphincter
  - Usually contains air
- Middle **body** Ⓙ
- Lower **pylorus** Ⓚ

Stomach Wall

- Similar to the intestinal wall (see Coloring Exercise 11-2)
- Three muscle layers to grind food and mix with digestive juices
  - **Longitudinal** Ⓛ
  - **Circular** Ⓜ
  - **Oblique** Ⓝ
- Inner layer (mucosa) folded into **rugae** Ⓞ when stomach is empty
- Between folds are **gastric pits** Ⓟ (gastric glands, see below), that secrete gastric juice

Gastric Pits

- Contain four epithelial cell types
  - **Mucous cells** Ⓠ: outer portion of pit
    - Secrete mucus to protect stomach
  - **Parietal cells** Ⓡ
    - Secrete **hydrochloric acid (HCl)** Ⓡ1
    - HCl destroys microbes, participates in protein digestion (below)
  - **Chief cells** Ⓢ
    - Secrete **pepsinogen** Ⓢ1 (see below)
  - **G cells** Ⓣ
    - Secrete gastrin into blood: regulates digestion

Protein Digestion

- HCl denatures **proteins** Ⓤ (straightens them out)
- HCl converts **pepsinogen** (Ⓢ1 inactive) into **pepsin** (Ⓢ2 active)
- Pepsin digests **proteins** Ⓤ into shorter **peptides** Ⓤ1

✎ **COLORING INSTRUCTIONS**

Color each structure and its name at the same time, using the same color. On the top figure:

1. Color the curved lines representing the stomach curvatures (Ⓐ and Ⓑ).

2. Color the esophagus Ⓒ and duodenum Ⓕ. Outline the circles representing the cardiac Ⓓ and pyloric orifices Ⓗ, and color the section of muscle forming the cardiac Ⓔ and pyloric Ⓗ sphincters.

3. Color the portions of the stomach wall that have not been cut away, representing the three stomach regions (Ⓘ to Ⓚ). Color the three layers of stomach muscle (Ⓛ to Ⓝ), and the inner surface folded into rugae Ⓞ.

✎ **COLORING INSTRUCTIONS**

On the bottom figure:

1. Lightly shade the rugae Ⓞ and gastric pit lumens Ⓟ.

2. Color the four cell types (Ⓠ to Ⓣ). Note that each cell type is shaped differently in this figure.

3. Go through the steps of protein digestion in the stomach, coloring the elements as you go.

4. Use related colors for the hydrogen ion (representing hydrochloric acid, Ⓡ1) and the parietal cell Ⓡ.

5. Use related colors for chief cells Ⓢ, the inactive pepsinogen Ⓢ1, and the active pepsin Ⓢ2.

6. Use related colors for proteins Ⓤ and peptides Ⓤ1.

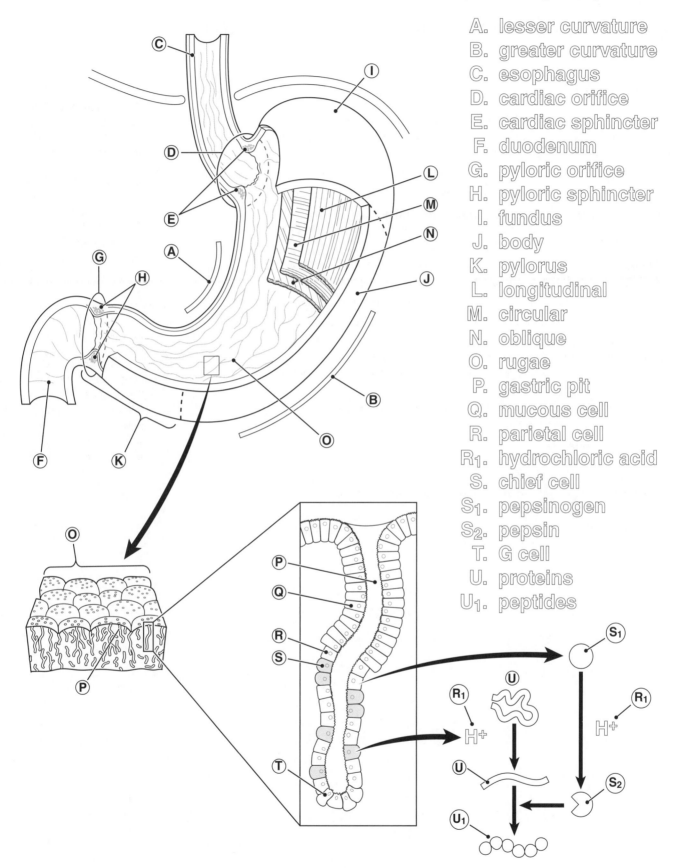

A. lesser curvature
B. greater curvature
C. esophagus
D. cardiac orifice
E. cardiac sphincter
F. duodenum
G. pyloric orifice
H. pyloric sphincter
I. fundus
J. body
K. pylorus
L. longitudinal
M. circular
N. oblique
O. rugae
P. gastric pit
Q. mucous cell
R. parietal cell
R_1. hydrochloric acid
S. chief cell
S_1. pepsinogen
S_2. pepsin
T. G cell
U. proteins
U_1. peptides

Coloring Exercise 11-5 ➤ Accessory Organs

Accessory Organs

- Produce and release secretions necessary for digestion
- Salivary glands (Coloring Exercise 11-1) release saliva into mouth (not shown)
- **Pancreas** Ⓐ and **liver** Ⓑ release secretions into **duodenum** Ⓒ

Pancreas Ⓐ

- Endocrine portion: synthesizes insulin/glucagon (Coloring Exercise 7-3)
- Exocrine portion: synthesizes **pancreatic juice** Ⓓ
  - Pancreatic enzymes: digest food (see Coloring Exercise 11-6)
  - Bicarbonate: neutralizes acidic gastric juices

Liver Ⓑ

- Functional cell: the hepatocyte
- Synthesizes blood proteins (albumin, transport proteins, clotting factors)
- Metabolizes hormones and drugs into less active forms
- Carbohydrate metabolism
  - Stores excess glucose in the form of glycogen
  - Converts glycogen and amino acids into glucose when required
- Fat metabolism
  - Generates ketones (used for energy) from fatty acids
  - Synthesizes lipoproteins
- Produces **bile** Ⓔ
  - Contains cholesterol
  - Contains bilirubin (waste product from degraded red blood cells)
  - Participates in fat processing (Coloring Exercise 11-6)
  - Stored in **gallbladder** Ⓕ
- Flow of bile and pancreatic juices illustrated in the bottom figure at right

COLORING INSTRUCTIONS

Color each structure and its name at the same time, using the same color. Color both figures together. As you color the structure in the top figure, lightly shade the box in the bottom figure.

1. Lightly shade the liver Ⓐ, pancreas Ⓑ, duodenum Ⓒ, and gallbladder Ⓕ.
2. Pancreatic juice Ⓓ and bile Ⓔ are represented by arrows on the bottom figure. Follow these secretions as they flow through different ducts (Ⓖ through Ⓛ).
3. Notice that one arrow is labeled both Ⓑ and Ⓓ, because it carries both bile and pancreatic juice.

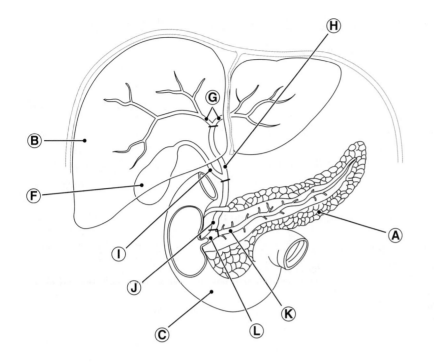

A. pancreas
B. liver
C. duodenum
D. pancreatic juice
E. bile
F. gallbladder
G. bile ducts
H. common hepatic duct
I. cystic duct
J. common bile duct
K. pancreatic duct
L. hepatopancreatic ampulla

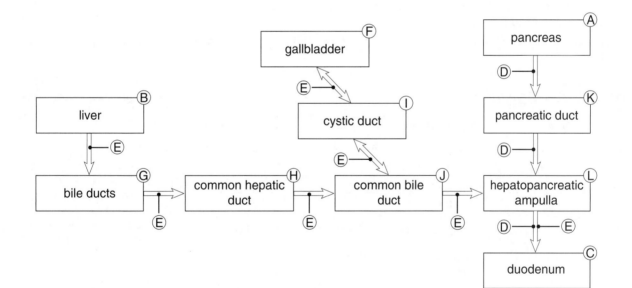

Coloring Exercise 11-6 ➤ Small Intestine: Digestion and Absorption

Fat Digestion

- Most dietary fat is in the form of **triglycerides** Ⓐ
  - Formed from **monoglyceride** Ⓑ + two **fatty acid** molecules Ⓒ
  - Triglycerides are hydrophobic; form large **droplets** Ⓐ1
    - Enzymes cannot access triglycerides in the middle of the droplet

Steps in Fat Digestion and Absorption

1. **Bile** Ⓓ emulsifies large **fat droplet** Ⓐ1 into many tiny fat droplets (**emulsion;** Ⓐ2)
   - Increases surface area; improves enzyme access
2. Pancreatic **lipase** Ⓔ digests **triglyceride** Ⓐ into **monoglyceride** Ⓑ and two **fatty acids** Ⓒ
3. Digestion products absorbed into **intestinal cell** Ⓕ
4. Monoglyceride and fatty acids reformed into triglycerides, then absorbed into lymph vessel (**lacteal** Ⓖ)

Protein Digestion

1. **Protein** Ⓗ digestion begins in the stomach (Coloring Exercise 11-4)
2. Pancreatic **trypsin** Ⓘ (and other enzymes) digest proteins into short **peptides** Ⓙ and **amino acids** Ⓚ
3. Short peptides and amino acids absorbed into **intestinal cells** Ⓕ, enter **blood vessels** Ⓛ

Carbohydrate Digestion

	Type	Composition	Enzyme	Enzyme Source
Starch Ⓜ	Polysaccharide	Long **glucose** Ⓝ chains	**Amylase** Ⓞ	Saliva and pancreas
Lactose Ⓟ	Disaccharide	**Glucose** Ⓝ+ **galactose** Ⓠ	**Lactase** Ⓡ	Intestinal cells
Maltose Ⓢ	Disaccharide	Two **glucose** Ⓝ	**Maltase** Ⓣ	Intestinal cells
Sucrose Ⓤ	Disaccharide	**Glucose** Ⓝ + **fructose** Ⓥ	**Sucrase** Ⓦ	Intestinal cells

Steps in Carbohydrate Digestion

1. Salivary amylase initiates starch digestion in mouth (not shown)
2. Pancreatic **amylase** Ⓞ digests starch to **maltose** Ⓡ in intestine
3. Enzymes in intestinal microvilli digest **disaccharides** (Ⓟ, Ⓢ, Ⓤ) to monosaccharides
4. Monosaccharides (**glucose** Ⓝ, **galactose** Ⓠ, **fructose** Ⓥ) absorbed by **intestinal cells** Ⓕ, enter **blood vessels** Ⓛ

✎ **COLORING INSTRUCTIONS**

Color each figure part and its name at the same time, using the same color.

1. Color the intestinal cells Ⓕ, lacteal Ⓖ, and blood vessels Ⓛ.
2. Follow the steps in fat digestion, coloring the different elements as you go (elements Ⓐ to Ⓔ).
3. Use the same color for Ⓐ, Ⓐ1 and Ⓐ2 (all are triglycerides).
4. Color the arrow representing the absorption of digested fats into the intestinal cell, using a mixture of colors used for Ⓑ and Ⓒ.
5. Color the second arrow, representing the absorption of newly formed triglycerides Ⓐ into the lacteal.

✎ **COLORING INSTRUCTIONS**

1. Follow the steps in protein digestion, coloring the different elements as you go (elements Ⓗ to Ⓛ).
2. Color the arrow representing the absorption of digested protein, using a mixture of colors used for Ⓙ and Ⓚ.

✎ **COLORING INSTRUCTIONS**

1. Follow the steps in carbohydrate digestion, coloring the different elements as you go (elements Ⓜ to Ⓦ).
2. Color the arrow representing the absorption of monosaccharides, using a mixture of colors used for Ⓝ, Ⓠ and Ⓥ.

A. triglyceride
A₁. fat droplet
A₂. emulsion
B. monoglyceride
C. fatty acid
D. bile
E. pancreatic lipase
F. intestinal cell

G. lacteal
H. protein
I. trypsin
J. peptides
K. amino acids
L. blood vessels
M. starch
N. glucose

O. amylase
P. lactose
Q. galactose
R. lactase
S. maltose
T. maltase
U. sucrose
V. fructose
W. sucrase

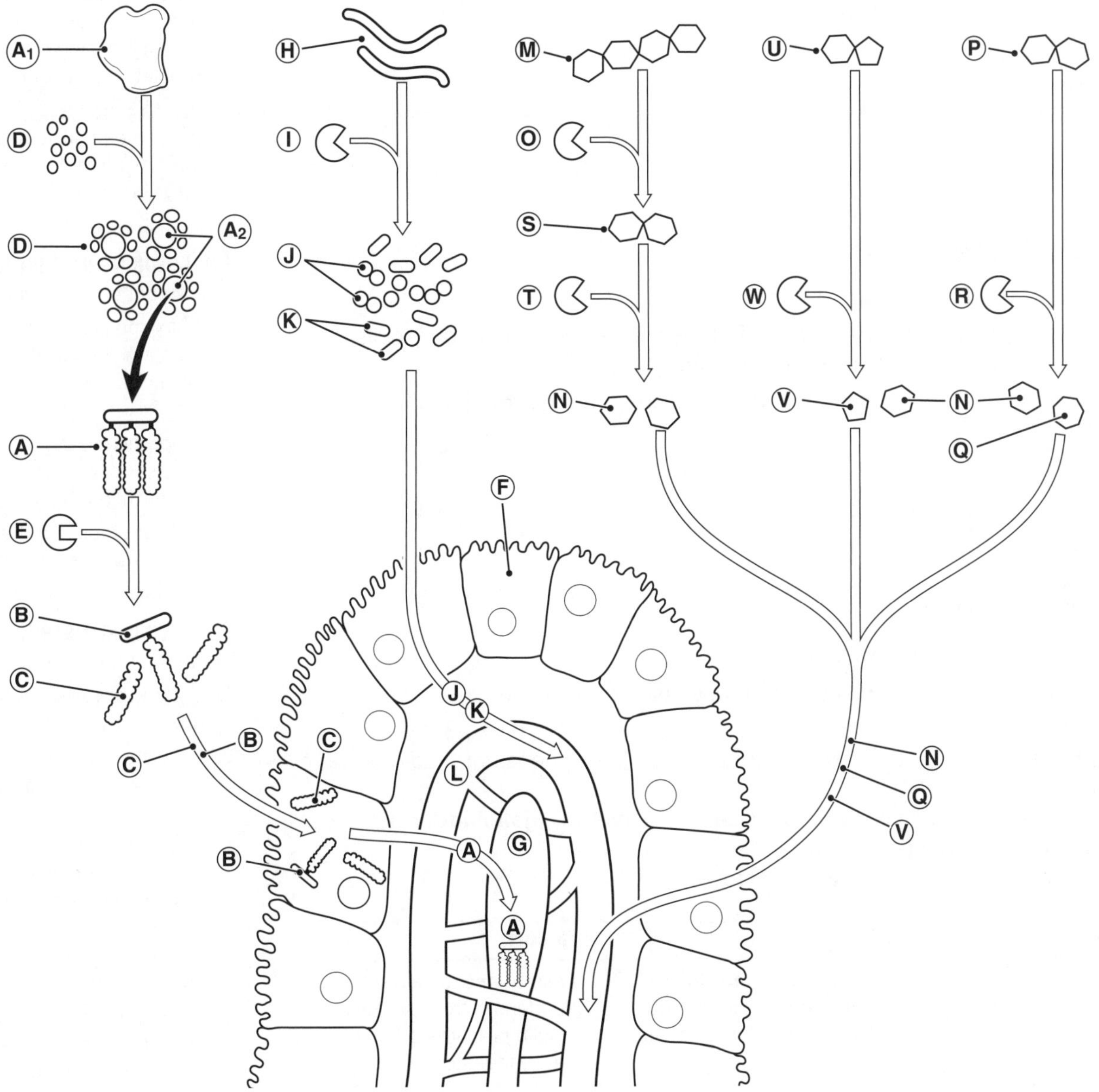

Coloring Exercise 11-7 ➤ Regulation of Digestion

Cephalic Phase

- Stimulus: thought, sight, smell of **food** Ⓐ
- Mediator: **nerves** Ⓑ to stomach
- Effect: **stimulates** Ⓒ **stomach motility** Ⓓ, secretion of **gastric juice** Ⓔ, saliva production (not shown)

COLORING INSTRUCTIONS

Color each structure and its name at the same time, using the same color. On the top left figure:

1. Color the cake Ⓐ and neuron Ⓑ.
2. Color the stomach wall, representing stomach motility Ⓓ, and the droplets, representing gastric secretions Ⓔ.
3. Color the positive sign Ⓒ, indicating that these functions are stimulated.

Gastric Phase

- Stimulus: **food** Ⓐ in stomach
- Mediator: **gastrin** Ⓕ (see Coloring Exercise 11-4) is synthesized by cells in stomach wall, released into **blood vessels** Ⓖ
- Effect: stimulates **stomach motility** Ⓓ, secretion of **gastric juice** Ⓔ

COLORING INSTRUCTIONS

On the bottom left figure:

1. Color the cake Ⓐ in the stomach (in real life the cake would no longer look like cake!).
2. Color the gastrin Ⓕ released from the stomach into blood Ⓖ.
3. Repeat steps 2 and 3 in the instructions above.

Intestinal Phase

- Stimulus: **food** Ⓐ in **duodenum** Ⓗ
- Mediators: nerves (not shown), hormones (see chart below)
- Effects:
  - **Inhibits** Ⓘ delivery of chyme from stomach (intestine is not ready for more food)
  - Increases secretion of digestive juices from **liver** Ⓙ, **gallbladder** Ⓚ, and **pancreas** Ⓛ into duodenum
  - Increases food digestion and absorption

COLORING INSTRUCTIONS

On the right-hand figure:

1. Color the cake Ⓐ in the duodenum Ⓗ.
2. Color the hormones secreted by the duodenum (Ⓜ, Ⓝ, Ⓟ) into the blood (blood not shown).
3. Color the stomach wall, representing stomach motility Ⓓ, and the droplets, representing gastric secretions Ⓔ.
4. Color the negative sign Ⓘ, indicating that gastric functions are inhibited.
5. Color the target organs of secretin and cholecystokinin, (Ⓙ, Ⓚ, Ⓛ) and the secretions of the target organs (Ⓞ, Ⓡ, Ⓞ).

Hormone	Action	Result
Gastric inhibitory peptide (GIP) Ⓜ	Reduces **gastric motility** Ⓓ and **secretion** Ⓔ; increased insulin secretion (not shown)	Less chyme is delivered to duodenum from stomach; insulin prepares body for newly ingested nutrients
Secretin Ⓝ	Increases secretion of pancreatic **bicarbonate** Ⓞ	Bicarbonate neutralizes acidic chyme, protecting duodenum
Cholecystokinin Ⓟ	Increases secretion of **bile** Ⓠ from **liver** Ⓙ and **gallbladder** Ⓚ; and of **pancreatic** Ⓡ **enzymes**	Bile emulsifies fat; pancreatic enzymes digest protein, starches, fats

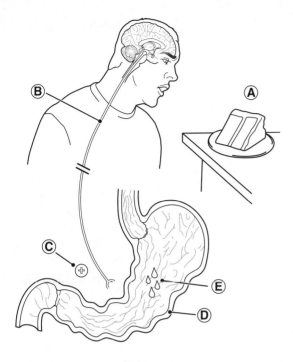

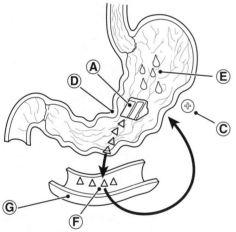

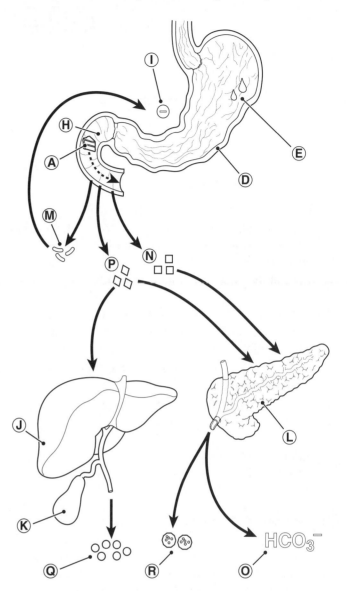

A. food
B. nerves
C. stimulation
D. stomach motility
E. gastric juice
F. gastrin
G. blood vessels

H. duodenum
I. inhibition
J. liver
K. gallbladder
L. pancreas
M. gastric inhibitory
    peptide

N. secretin
O. bicarbonate
P. cholecystokinin
Q. bile
R. pancreatic
    enzymes

CHAPTER 12

The Urinary System and Water Balance

Coloring Exercise 12-1 ➤ Water Balance

Fluid Compartments

- **Water** Ⓐ makes up 60% of body weight
- Extracellular fluid (outside of cells): 20% of body weight
  - **Plasma, lymph** Ⓑ: 5% of body weight
  - **Interstitial fluid** (between cells) Ⓒ: 15% of body weight
- **Intracellular fluid** Ⓓ (within cells): 40% of body weight

Fluid Exchanges Between Compartments

- Fluid moves between **plasma/lymph** Ⓑ and **interstitial fluid** Ⓒ by crossing the endothelial layer of blood and lymphatic **capillaries** Ⓔ
- Fluid moves between the **interstitial fluid** Ⓒ and the **intracellular fluid** Ⓓ by crossing the **plasma membrane** Ⓕ
- Fluid enters the blood from the **intestines** Ⓖ
- Fluid leaves the blood via the:
  - **intestines** Ⓖ
  - **skin** Ⓗ (sweating)
  - **lungs** Ⓘ (water vapor)
  - **kidneys** Ⓙ (urine)

Water Gain and Loss

- Water gain should equal water loss
  - Loss > gain = electrolyte imbalances, dehydration
  - Gain > loss = electrolyte imbalances, bloating
  - Average volumes gained and lost are listed below
- Sources of water gain
  - **Metabolism** Ⓚ: 200 ml
    - water is a byproduct of metabolic reactions
    - e.g., glucose breakdown to generate ATP
    - water added directly to intracellular fluid
  - **Food** Ⓛ: 700 mL (varies widely)
  - **Drink** Ⓜ: 1600 mL (varies widely)
- Sources of water loss
  - **Feces** Ⓝ: 200 mL
  - **Lungs** Ⓘ: 300 mL
  - **Skin** Ⓗ: 500 mL
  - **Urine** Ⓞ: 1500 mL (varies widely)
- Body regulates water loss in urine and dietary water gain
  - Water gain: dehydration stimulates thirst
  - Water loss: dehydration reduces urine production (Coloring Exercise 12-5)

COLORING INSTRUCTIONS

Color each figure part and its name at the same time, using the same color. On the top figure:

1. Color the fluid compartments (Ⓐ to Ⓓ), beginning with the small body. The volume of fluid in the compartment is proportional to the percentage of body weight.
2. Color the tubes connecting the different compartments, representing capillary endothelial cells Ⓔ and plasma membranes Ⓕ.
3. Color the organs involved in fluid balance (Ⓖ to Ⓙ).

COLORING INSTRUCTIONS

On the bottom figure:

1. Color the boxes representing water gained and lost. Note that the box size is proportional to the volumes listed in the narrative.
2. For food Ⓛ, drink Ⓜ, and feces Ⓝ, use colors similar to the color used above for the intestines Ⓖ.
3. For urine Ⓞ, use a color similar to the one used above for the kidney Ⓙ.

A. water
B. plasma, lymph
C. interstitial fluid
D. intracelluar fluid
E. capillary
   endothelium
F. plasma membrane
G. intestines
H. skin
 I. lungs
J. kidneys
K. metabolism
L. food
M. drink
N. feces
O. urine

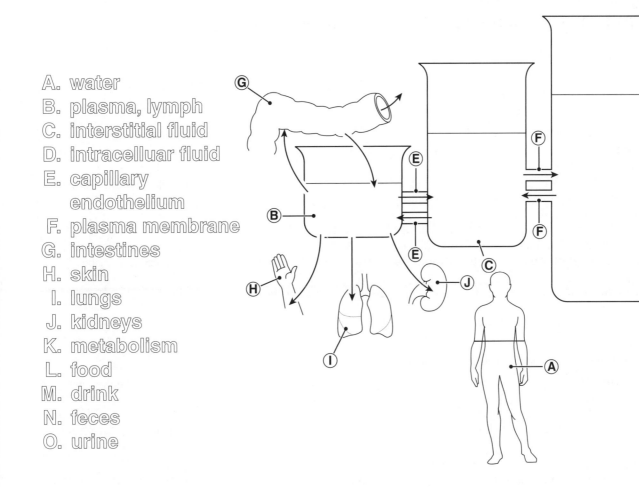

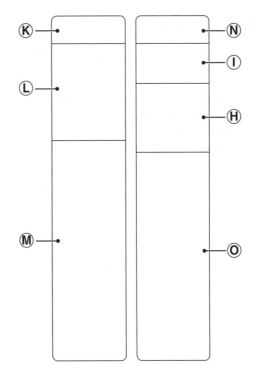

Coloring Exercise 12-2 ➤ The Urinary System

Organs of the Urinary System

- **Kidneys** Ⓐ
  - Form urine, containing
    - Excess water
    - Metabolic wastes (e.g., urea)
    - Excess acid
    - Excess electrolytes (e.g., sodium)
  - Produce hormones that regulate
    - Red blood cell synthesis (erythropoietin: Coloring Exercise 8-3)
    - Water balance (renin: Coloring Exercise 12-6)
  - Receive **arterial blood** Ⓑ① from the **abdominal aorta** Ⓑ via the **renal artery** Ⓒ
  - **Venous blood** Ⓔ① from kidney drains into **renal vein** Ⓓ and the **inferior vena cava** Ⓔ
  - **Adrenal glands** Ⓕ (Coloring Exercise 7-7) lie atop of both kidneys
- **Ureters** Ⓖ
  - Drain **urine** Ⓗ from kidney into urinary bladder
- **Urinary bladder** Ⓘ
  - Urine reservoir
  - Lined with transitional epithelium (Coloring Exercise 1-7)
  - Expands to hold about 470 mL of urine
- **Urethra** Ⓙ
  - Conducts urine from bladder outside the body
  - In males, the **prostate gland** Ⓚ surrounds the urethra

The Kidney: Gross Anatomy

- Surrounded by a **capsule** Ⓛ of fibrous connective tissue
  - Indentation where vessels and the ureters attach is called the **hilum** Ⓜ
- Consists of outer **cortex** Ⓝ and inner **medulla** Ⓞ
  - Medulla contains darker regions called **pyramids** Ⓟ
- Urine produced by kidney tissue drains into renal calyces (singular, **calyx** Ⓠ) and then into the **renal pelvis** Ⓡ
  - Some calyces contain **fat** Ⓢ
  - Renal pelvis drains into the **ureter** Ⓖ

🖊 COLORING INSTRUCTIONS

Color each structure and its name at the same time, using the same color. On the top figure:

1. Color the renal veins Ⓓ and the renal arteries Ⓒ medium blue and medium red, respectively.

2. Color the aorta Ⓑ and its branches (not labeled) light red. Color the arrow representing arterial blood flow Ⓑ① dark red.

3. Color the inferior vena cava Ⓔ and its branches (not labeled) light blue. Color the arrow representing venous blood flow Ⓔ① dark blue.

4. Color the organs of the urinary system (Ⓖ, Ⓘ, Ⓙ) and related organs (Ⓕ and Ⓚ).

5. Color the arrows representing urine flow Ⓗ yellow.

🖊 COLORING INSTRUCTIONS

On the bottom figure:

1. Color the renal capsule Ⓛ. Use a dark color to outline the circles representing the kidney hilum Ⓜ.

2. Lightly shade the renal cortex Ⓝ and the entire renal medulla Ⓞ using contrasting colors. A dotted line surrounds the renal medulla.

3. Use a darker version of the color used for the medulla to color the pyramids Ⓟ.

4. Color the renal calyces Ⓠ and the renal pelvis Ⓡ. A dotted line indicates the separation between these two structures.

5. Color the ureter Ⓖ, renal artery (and tributaries) Ⓒ, and renal vein (and tributaries) Ⓓ.

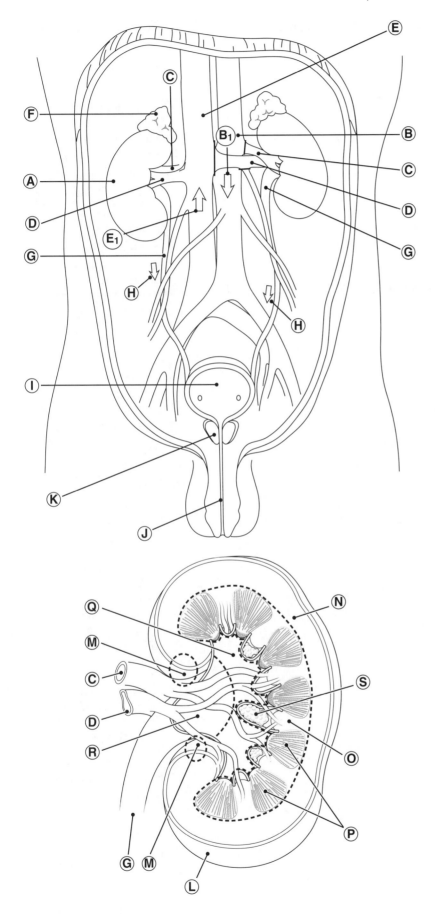

A. kidney
B. abdominal aorta
B_1. arterial blood flow
C. renal artery
D. renal vein
E. inferior vena cava
E_1. venous blood flow
F. adrenal gland
G. ureter
H. urine
I. urinary bladder
J. urethra
K. prostate gland
L. capsule
M. hilum
N. cortex
O. medulla
P. pyramids
Q. calyx
R. renal pelvis
S. fat

Coloring Exercise 12-3 ➤ The Nephron and Its Blood Supply

The Nephron

- Tiny, coiled tube; the basic unit of the kidney
- Exchanges substances with blood using filtration, diffusion, osmosis, and active transport (see Coloring Exercises 1-6 and 12-4)
- Fluid found in nephrons is called filtrate

Parts of the Nephron

Filtrate passes through the nephron as follows:

1. **Glomerular capsule** Ⓐ
2. **Proximal convoluted tubule** Ⓑ
3. **Loop of Henle** (**descending** Ⓒ and **ascending** Ⓓ limbs)
4. **Distal convoluted tubule** Ⓔ
5. **Collecting duct** Ⓕ
6. **Calyx** Ⓖ and renal pelvis (not shown)

Blood Supply

- Each nephron associated with two capillary beds
  - **Glomerulus** Ⓚ: generates filtrate (see Coloring Exercise 12-4)
  - **Peritubular capillaries** Ⓜ: exchange substances with filtrate (see Coloring Exercise 12-4)
- Blood passes through the renal vessels as shown below

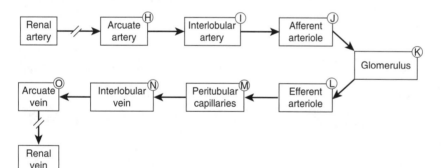

COLORING INSTRUCTIONS

Color each structure and its name at the same time, using the same color.

1. Color the parts of the nephron (Ⓐ to Ⓔ) in top figure, in which most of the vessels have been removed.
2. Color the nephron parts Ⓐ to Ⓖ on bottom figure.
3. Use variants of yellow, orange, and brown.

COLORING INSTRUCTIONS

1. Follow blood flowing through the kidney on the flowchart and the figure.
2. Use variants of red for the arteries (Ⓗ to Ⓙ, Ⓛ) variants of purple for the capillary beds (Ⓚ, Ⓜ), and variants of blue for the veins (Ⓝ, Ⓞ).
3. Color the vessel(s) on the diagram and the relevant box on the flowchart using the same color.
4. Note that the renal artery and renal vein are not shown in the drawing. There are a number of other vessels between the renal vessels and the arcuate vessels, as indicated by the break in the arrow.

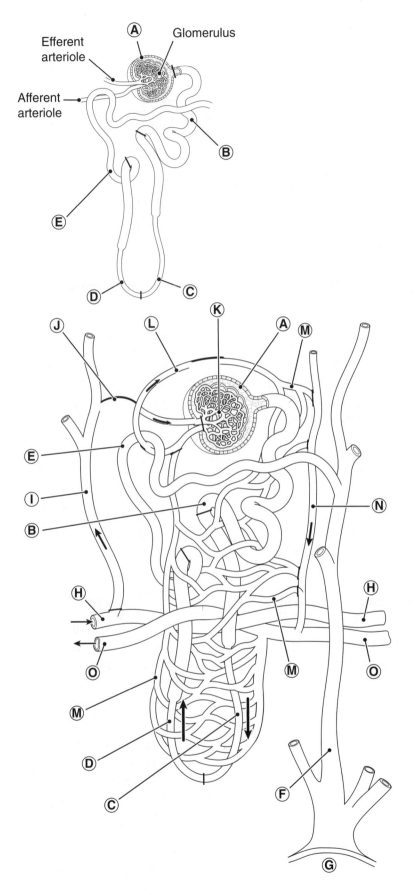

A. glomerular capsule
B. proximal convoluted tubule
C. descending loop of Henle
D. ascending loop of Henle
E. distal convoluted tubule
F. collecting duct
G. calyx
H. arcuate artery
 I. interlobular artery
J. afferent arteriole
K. glomerulus
L. efferent arteriole
M. peritubular capillaries
N. interlobular vein
O. arcuate vein

Efferent arteriole

Glomerulus

Afferent arteriole

Coloring Exercise 12-4 ➤ Urine Formation

Filtration

- Note that the entry to the **glomerulus** Ⓐ (**afferent arteriole** Ⓑ) is larger than the exit (**efferent arteriole** Ⓒ)
  - Blood in glomerular capillaries is under high pressure (think of partially blocking the end of a garden hose with your finger)
  - Water and **soluble molecules** Ⓓ are forced through the capillary **endothelium** Ⓔ into the **glomerular capsule** Ⓕ
  - Resulting fluid is called the **filtrate** Ⓖ, containing nutrients (glucose, amino acids), ions, urea, vitamins, drugs, and other solutes
  - **Red blood cells** Ⓗ and **proteins** Ⓘ are too large to fit between endothelial cells; retained in the blood
  - Entire plasma volume (3.5 L) is filtered every 30 minutes
  - Filtrate passes down **proximal convoluted tubule** Ⓙ

Urine Formation

- Urine formation involves exchanges between renal capillary beds (the **glomerulus** Ⓐ and the **peritubular capillaries** Ⓚ) and the nephron
- Involves three processes: **filtration** Ⓛ, **reabsorption** Ⓜ, and **secretion** Ⓝ

Filtration Ⓛ
- Occurs between the **glomerulus** Ⓐ and the **glomerular capsule** Ⓕ
- Produces filtrate; discussed above

Reabsorption Ⓜ
- Substances move from the **filtrate** Ⓖ into the **peritubular capillaries** Ⓚ
- Reabsorbed substances are NOT excreted in urine
- Water, amino acids, glucose, sodium, potassium, and hydrogen are reabsorbed by diffusion, active transport, osmosis
- **Water reabsorption** Ⓞ in the distal tubule is regulated by ADH (see Coloring Exercise 12-7)

Secretion Ⓝ
- Substances move from the **peritubular capillaries** Ⓚ into the **filtrate** Ⓖ
- Potassium and hydrogen ions are frequently secreted
- Some secreted substances are reabsorbed into the blood
- Secreted substances that are not reabsorbed are excreted in urine

---

✎ COLORING INSTRUCTIONS

Color each figure part and its name at the same time, using the same color. On the top figure:

1. Use the same colors as in Coloring Exercise 12-3 to color the afferent Ⓑ and efferent Ⓒ arterioles and the four uncut capillaries shown for the glomerulus Ⓐ. Shade VERY LIGHTLY the glomerular capillary that has been cut open.

2. Use a dark color to outline the capillary endothelial cells Ⓔ lining the cut-open capillary.

3. Use contrasting dark colors for the proteins (diamonds, Ⓘ) and blood cells (circles, Ⓗ) that stay in the glomerular capillary.

4. Lightly shade the filtrate Ⓖ yellow. Use darker variants of yellow for the walls of the glomerular capsule Ⓕ and the proximal convoluted tubule Ⓙ.

5. Color the solute molecules (triangles, Ⓓ) in the blood and filtrate.

✎ COLORING INSTRUCTIONS

On the bottom figure:

1. Color the afferent Ⓑ and efferent Ⓒ arterioles, the glomerulus Ⓐ, and the peritubular capillaries Ⓚ.

2. Lightly shade the glomerular capsule Ⓕ and the filtrate Ⓖ passing down the nephron.

3. Color the four arrows representing filtration Ⓛ, reabsorption Ⓜ, secretion Ⓝ, and ADH-regulated water reabsorption Ⓞ.

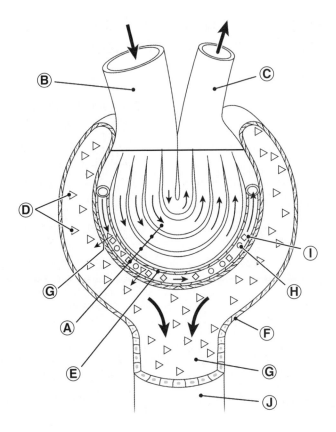

A. glomerulus
B. afferent arteriole
C. efferent arteriole
D. soluble molecules
E. endothelium
F. glomerular capsule
G. filtrate
H. red blood cells
I. proteins
J. proximal convoluted
tubule
K. peritubular capillaries
L. filtration
M. reabsorption
N. secretion
O. ADH-dependent
water reabsorption

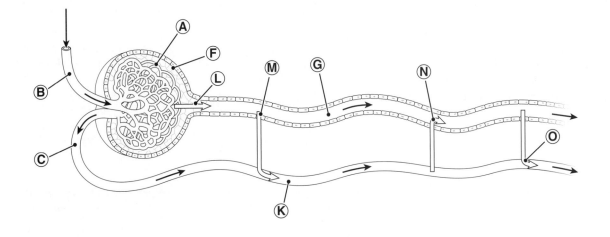

Coloring Exercise 12-5 ➤ Regulation of Renal Function: ADH and Urine Concentration

Concentrated Urine Generation

- Water moves by osmosis (see Coloring Exercise 1-6)
  - Osmolarity = overall concentration of solutes in a fluid
  - **Water** Ⓐ moves from area of lower osmolarity (less solute, more water) to area of higher osmolarity (more solute, less water)
- **Interstitial fluid** Ⓑ osmolarity: low in cortex (top of diagram), high in medulla
- **Filtrate** Ⓒ osmolarity: if possible, it will match the interstitial fluid osmolarity

Changes in Filtrate Osmolarity

- **Proximal tubule** Ⓓ: 300 mOsm (dilute)
- **Descending loop of Henle** Ⓔ: osmolarity increases
  - **Aquaporins** Ⓕ (water channels) are present
  - As **filtrate** Ⓒ moves down loop, it encounters more concentrated **interstitial fluid** Ⓑ (higher osmolarity)
  - **Water** Ⓐ leaves filtrate by osmosis
- **Ascending loop of Henle** Ⓖ: osmolarity decreases
  - No aquaporins: no water movement
  - **Sodium pumps** Ⓗ: actively pump **sodium** Ⓘ out of filtrate
  - Less sodium = less filtrate osmolarity
- **Distal tubule** Ⓙ and **collecting duct** Ⓚ
  - **Aquaporins** Ⓕ are present ONLY if antidiuretic hormone (**ADH** Ⓛ) is present
  - ADH is discussed in Coloring Exercises 7-4 and 12-6
  - If ADH is present
    - **Water** Ⓐ leaves **filtrate** Ⓒ by osmosis as it descends the collecting duct
    - Filtrate leaves collecting duct deep in the medulla, where interstitial fluid is very concentrated
    - A small volume of concentrated **urine** Ⓜ is produced
  - If ADH is not present,
    - Aquaporins are not present
    - Water cannot leave the collecting duct
    - Large volume of dilute **urine** Ⓜ is produced

✍ **COLORING INSTRUCTIONS**

Color each figure part and its name at the same time, using the same color.
On the top figure:

1. Color the walls of the different sections of the nephron (Ⓓ, Ⓔ, Ⓖ, Ⓙ, Ⓚ). Do not color the interior.

2. Use blue to color the arrow and three numbers indicating the interstitial fluid osmolarity Ⓑ. Vary the intensity of the color in accordance with the fluid osmolarity.

3. Color the numbers INSIDE the nephron Ⓒ yellow, representing filtrate osmolarity. Color the filtrate Ⓒ in the nephron yellow.

4. Color the aquaporins Ⓕ and the arrows representing water movement Ⓐ, and the sodium pumps Ⓗ and the arrows representing sodium movement Ⓘ.

5. Color ADH Ⓛ, and the small volume of urine Ⓜ produced when ADH is present.

6. Follow the filtrate through the nephron, noting how water and sodium movement change the osmolarity.

✍ **COLORING INSTRUCTIONS**

On the bottom figure:

1. Follow steps 2–3 above, and color the wall of the collecting duct Ⓚ.

2. Color the ADH Ⓛ symbol, noting the X that signifies the absence of ADH.

3. Color the large volume of dilute urine Ⓜ produced when ADH is absent.

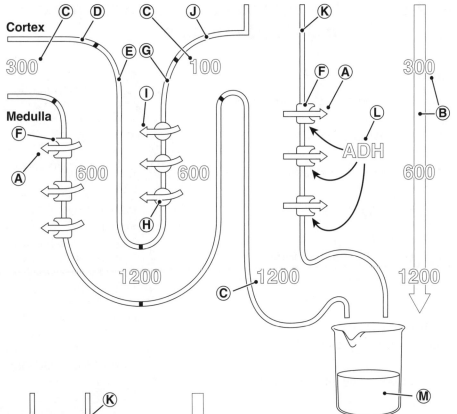

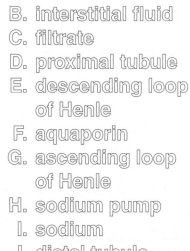

A. water
B. interstitial fluid
C. filtrate
D. proximal tubule
E. descending loop of Henle
 F. aquaporin
G. ascending loop of Henle
H. sodium pump
 I. sodium
J. distal tubule
K. collecting tubule
L. ADH
M. urine

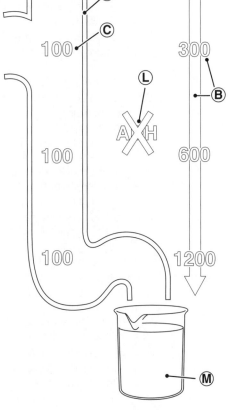

Coloring Exercise 12-6 ➤ The Juxtaglomerular Apparatus and Blood Pressure

The Juxtaglomerular Apparatus

- Consists of cells of the **afferent arteriole** Ⓑ and cells of the **distal tubule** Ⓒ
- Measures filtrate flow in the distal tubule
  - Remember that the blood pressure drives filtration
  - Lower blood pressure = less filtration = less filtrate
- Secretes **renin** Ⓓ when flow (and thus blood pressure) is low

The Renin-Angiotensin-Aldosterone System

- Powerful system for increasing blood pressure
- Involves three active hormones: **angiotensin II** Ⓔ, **aldosterone** Ⓕ, **antidiuretic hormone** Ⓖ

Production of Angiotensin II

1. **Low blood pressure** Ⓗ stimulates **renin** Ⓓ production
2. Renin (an enzyme) cleaves **angiotensinogen** Ⓘ (produced by **liver** Ⓙ) into **angiotensin I** Ⓚ
3. **Angiotensin converting enzyme** Ⓛ (produced by **lungs** Ⓜ) cleaves angiotensin I to **angiotensin II** Ⓔ

Actions of Angiotensin II (ATII)

- ATII acts at **hypothalamus** Ⓝ to
  - Stimulate **thirst** Ⓞ
  - Stimulate **cardiac output** Ⓟ and **vasoconstriction** Ⓠ
  - Stimulate **antidiuretic hormone** Ⓖ production
    - ADH released by posterior pituitary (not shown)
    - ADH increases **water retention** Ⓡ (Coloring Exercise 12-5); decreases urine output
- ATII acts at **adrenal cortex** Ⓢ
  - Stimulates **aldosterone** production Ⓕ
  - Aldosterone acts on **kidney** Ⓣ to increase **salt reabsorption** Ⓤ (and, indirectly, water reabsorption)

Net Result

- Increased cardiac output and vasoconstriction → **increased blood pressure** Ⓥ
- Increased blood volume (more water intake, less water in urine) → increased blood pressure

✍ **COLORING INSTRUCTIONS**

Color each figure part and its name at the same time, using the same color. On the top figure:

1. Save dark red and bright green for later.
2. Color the afferent arteriole Ⓑ and the distal tubule Ⓒ on both diagrams.
3. Color in the small box outlining the cells of the juxtaglomerular apparatus Ⓐ.
4. If you like, you can color the rest of the nephron light yellow, and the other blood vessels light red.

✍ **COLORING INSTRUCTIONS**

On the bottom figure:

1. Color the symbols representing low blood pressure Ⓗ dark red, the small drawing of the juxtaglomerular apparatus Ⓐ, and the renin molecules Ⓓ.
2. Color the angiotensinogen molecule Ⓘ produced by the liver Ⓙ, and the angiotensin I Ⓚ molecule resulting from renin action. Note the relative length of the two molecules.
3. Color the ACE enzyme Ⓛ produced by the lungs Ⓜ, and the angiotensin II Ⓔ molecule resulting from ACE action.
4. Color the target sites for angiotensin II (Ⓝ Ⓢ) and cartoons representing direct actions (Ⓞ to Ⓠ).
5. Color the names of hormones (Ⓕ and Ⓖ) produced in response to AT II.
6. Color the kidney Ⓣ and the symbols representing aldosterone actions at the kidney (Ⓤ Ⓡ).
7. Finally, use green to color the symbols representing increased blood pressure Ⓥ.

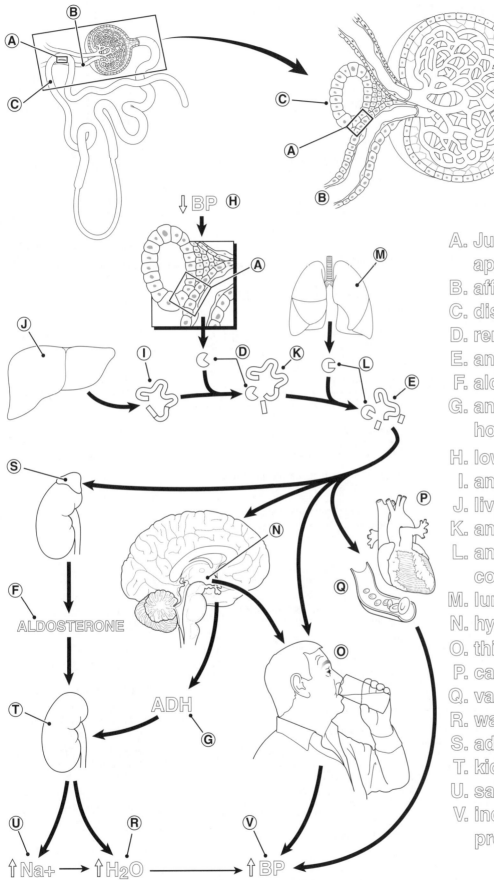

Ⓐ low BP Ⓗ

A. Juxtaglomerular
   apparatus
B. afferent arteriole
C. distal tubule
D. renin
E. angiotensin II
F. aldosterone
G. antidiuretic
   hormone
H. low blood pressure
 I. angiotensinogen
J. liver
K. antiogensin I
L. angiotensin
   converting enzyme
M. lungs
N. hypothalamus
O. thirst
 P. cardiac output
Q. vasoconstriction
R. water retention
S. adrenal cortex
T. kidney
U. salt reabsorption
V. increased blood
   pressure

ALDOSTERONE

ADH

⇑Na+ ⟶ ⇑H₂O ⟶ ⇑BP

Coloring Exercise 12-7 ➤ Urinalysis

Urinalysis

- Urine sample analyzed chemically, using a "**dipstick**" Ⓐ
- Urine sediment analyzed microscopically
  - Casts: mass of material, most types indicate disease

	Normal Finding	Abnormal Findings (examples)
Dipstick Analysis		
Glucose Ⓑ	Absent	Present: diabetes mellitus
Bilirubin Ⓒ	Absent	Present: jaundice (liver disease)
Ketones Ⓓ	Absent	Present: diabetes mellitus
Specific gravity Ⓔ	1.016–1.022 (indicates concentration of dissolved solutes)	Increased: dehydration Decreased: excessive fluid intake (often alcohol), diabetes insipidus
Blood Ⓕ (see below)	Absent	Present: anemia, renal disease
pH Ⓖ	About 6 (acidic)	Less acidic: vegetarian diet, bacterial contamination More acidic: respiratory or metabolic dysfunction
Protein Ⓗ (see below)	Absent	Present: vigorous exercise, fever, sometimes renal disease
Urobilinogen Ⓘ	Small amounts	Large amounts: jaundice
Nitrite Ⓙ	Absent	Present: urinary tract infection (produced by bacteria)
Leukocyte esterase Ⓚ	Absent	Present: urinary tract infection (produced by bacteria)
Visual and Microscopic Analysis		
Appearance Ⓛ	Clear, light yellow	Cloudy: infection Red: intact or destroyed blood cells (or beets!) Brown: jaundice
Odor	Odorless	Ketone odor: diabetes mellitus Foul odor: bacterial contamination of sample
Protein casts Ⓜ	None	Present: renal disease
White cell casts Ⓝ	None	Present: infection
Red cell casts Ⓞ	None	Present: disease of the glomerulus
Red blood cells Ⓟ	Few	Numerous: bleeding in urinary tract (or specimen contamination)
White blood cells Ⓠ	Few	Numerous: infection or specimen contamination
Bacteria Ⓡ	None	Present: infection
Crystals Ⓢ	Some	Many: hypercalcemia
Epithelial cells Ⓣ	Few	Many: infection, inflammation, malignancy

✎ **COLORING INSTRUCTIONS**

Color each figure part and its name at the same time, using the same color.
On the top figure:

1. Color the top part of the dipstick Ⓐ and the squares (Ⓑ to Ⓚ), used to detect different substances in urine.
2. Color the urine sample Ⓛ, which is evaluated for color and clarity.

✎ **COLORING INSTRUCTIONS**

On the bottom figure: Color the different substances that are observed microscopically in normal and abnormal urine (Ⓜ to Ⓣ).

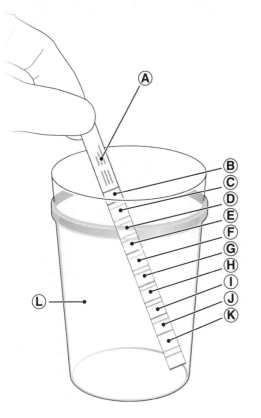

A. dipstick
B. glucose
C. bilirubin
D. ketones
E. specific gravity
F. blood
G. pH
H. protein
I. urobilinogen
J. nitrate
K. leukocyte esterase
L. appearance
M. protein casts
N. white cell casts
O. red cell casts
P. red blood cells
Q. white blood cells
R. bacteria
S. crystals
T. epithelial cells

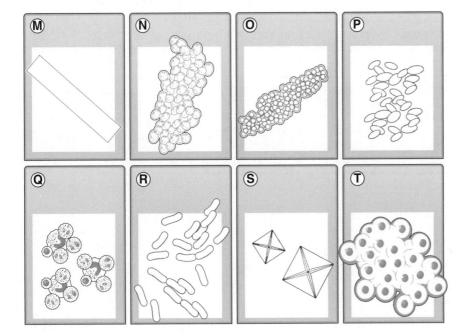

Reproduction and Heredity

Coloring Exercise 13-1 ➤ The Male Reproductive System

	Structure	Function
Testis Ⓐ	Large gland (see Coloring Exercise 13-2)	Synthesizes testosterone and spermatozoa
Scrotum Ⓑ	Sac containing testes; located outside the body	Maintains testicular temperature lower than the rest of the body
Epididymis Ⓒ	Long, coiled tube at the posterior of the testes	Site of sperm maturation and storage
Ductus deferens Ⓓ	Narrow, stiff, muscular tube; enlarged end portion (**ampulla** Ⓔ) located ventrally to **rectum** Ⓕ	Conducts sperm from **epididymis** Ⓒ to **ejaculatory duct** Ⓗ
Seminal vesicles Ⓖ	Exocrine glands	Produce thick, yellow, sugary, alkaline secretion to nourish sperm (part of semen)
Ejaculatory duct Ⓗ	Union of seminal vesicle duct and ductus deferens	Conducts sperm and seminal vesicle secretions to urethra
Urethra Ⓘ	Tube extending from **bladder** Ⓙ to end of penis (the **ureter** Ⓛ conveys urine from **kidney** Ⓜ to bladder)	Conveys urine and semen out of body
Penis Ⓚ	See below; end covered by the **prepuce** Ⓚ1 in uncircumcised males	Permits sexual intercourse; contains urethra
Bulbourethral gland Ⓝ	Small pea-sized exocrine gland	Secretes mucus to facilitate sexual intercourse
Prostate Ⓞ	Encircles urethra	Produces thin, alkaline secretion (part of semen) to neutralize acidity of female reproductive tract

📝 COLORING INSTRUCTIONS

Color each structure and its name at the same time, using the same color. On the larger figure:

1. Color all structures except for Ⓚ, Ⓚ1, Ⓢ, and Ⓣ. Save a red, a blue, and a yellow for later.

2. Only color the skin of the scrotum Ⓑ.

3. Use black to draw the arrows representing the pathway of sperm. Some of the arrows have already been drawn for you.

📝 COLORING INSTRUCTIONS

On both figures:

1. Color the skin of the penis Ⓚ. Use a related color for the prepuce Ⓚ1.

2. Color the internal parts of the penis. Use red for arteries Ⓟ, blue for veins Ⓠ, and yellow for the nerve Ⓡ. Use related colors for the corpus spongiosum Ⓣ and the glans penis Ⓤ.

Structure of the Penis

- Contains spongy (erectile) tissue
  - Fills with blood during erection
    - **Arterial** Ⓟ smooth muscle relaxes, enabling blood to flow in
    - **Venous** Ⓠ smooth muscle contracts, preventing blood from leaving
    - Erection controlled by **nerves** Ⓡ
  - **Corpus cavernosa** Ⓢ
    - Two columns of erectile tissue
  - **Corpus spongiosum** Ⓣ
    - Contains the **urethra** Ⓘ
    - Enlarges at the end to form the **glans penis** Ⓤ

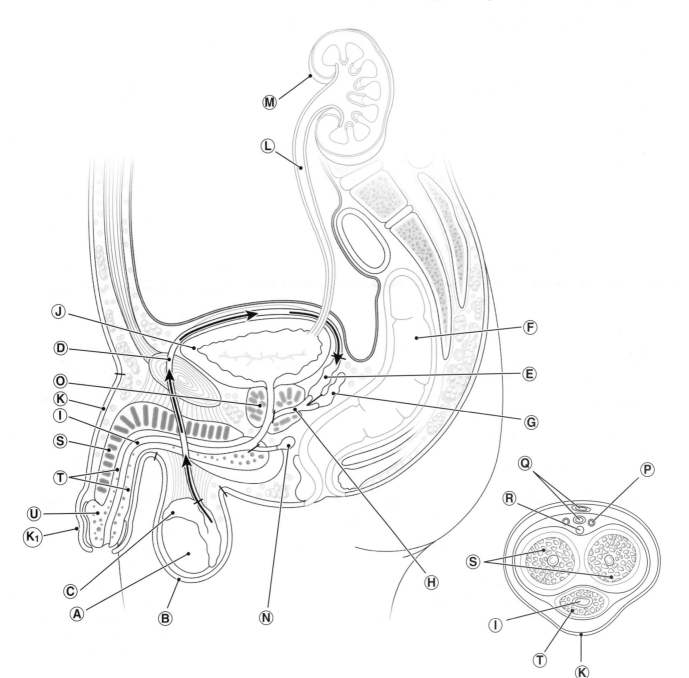

A. testis
B. scrotum
C. epididymis
D. ductus deferens
E. ampulla
F. rectum
G. seminal vesicles
H. ejaculatory duct

I. urethra
J. bladder
K. penis
K₁. prepuce
L. ureter
M. kidney
N. bulbourethral
   gland

O. prostate
P. arteries
Q. veins
R. nerve
S. corpus cavernosa
T. corpus spongiosum
U. glans penis

Coloring Exercise 13-2 ➤ The Testis and Spermatogenesis

Anatomy of the Testis and Scrotum

- **Testis** (A)
  - Protected by connective tissue **capsule** (B)
  - Extensions of capsule (**septum** (B1), or septa (plural)) divide testis into **lobules** (A1)
  - Each lobule contains **seminiferous tubules** (C) (see below)
  - Seminiferous tubules drain into the **rete testis** (D), then into the **efferent ducts** (E), and subsequently into the **epididymal duct** (F) of the epididymis
- **Epididymis** (G): looks like a "comma" on the posterior portion of the testis
  - Consists of a **head** (G1) and a **body** (G2)
- **Spermatic cord** (H): joins scrotum to body
  - Contains **testicular artery** (I), **veins** (J), **nerves** (K), **ductus deferens** (L), and lymphatic vessels (not shown)

Seminiferous Tubules

- **Interstitial cells** (M): located BETWEEN seminiferous tubules
  - Synthesize testosterone
  - Regulated by luteinizing hormone from the anterior pituitary gland
- **Sustentacular cells** (N) (also called Sertoli or nurse cells)
  - Large cells; easily identifiable nucleus
  - Secrete testosterone binding protein
  - Nourish and protect developing gametes
    - Gametes develop between adjacent cells
- Gametes
  - **Spermatogonium** (O): sperm precursor cells (stem cells)
    - Divides by mitosis to produce one spermatogonium and one primary spermatocyte
  - **Primary spermatocyte** (P) divides to produce two secondary spermatocytes (23 chromosomes each)
  - Each **secondary spermatocyte** (Q) divides to produce two spermatids
  - **Spermatids** (R) mature into **spermatozoa** (S)

✍ COLORING INSTRUCTIONS

Color each figure part and its name at the same time, using the same color. On the top figure:

1. Dotted lines divide the testis (A), the epididymis (G), and the spermatic cord (H). LIGHTLY shade over these three compartments, so that the structures within them remain visible, using the same color for the epididymis head (G1) and body (G2).

2. Use the same color for the capsule (B) and the septa (B1). Do not color the lobules (A1).

3. Use related colors to outline the seminiferous tubules (C), the rete testis (D), and the efferent ducts (E).

4. Use a contrasting dark color for the epididymal duct (F).

5. Color the ductus deferens (L), veins (J), artery (I), and nerve (K) in the spermatic cord.

✍ COLORING INSTRUCTIONS

On the bottom figure:

1. On the small locator figure, color the entire seminiferous tubule (C) using the same color as above.

2. The larger figure shows the cells resulting from one round of cell division beginning from one spermatogonium. Color the large sustentacular cells (N), the interstitial cells (M) and the developing gametes (O to S).

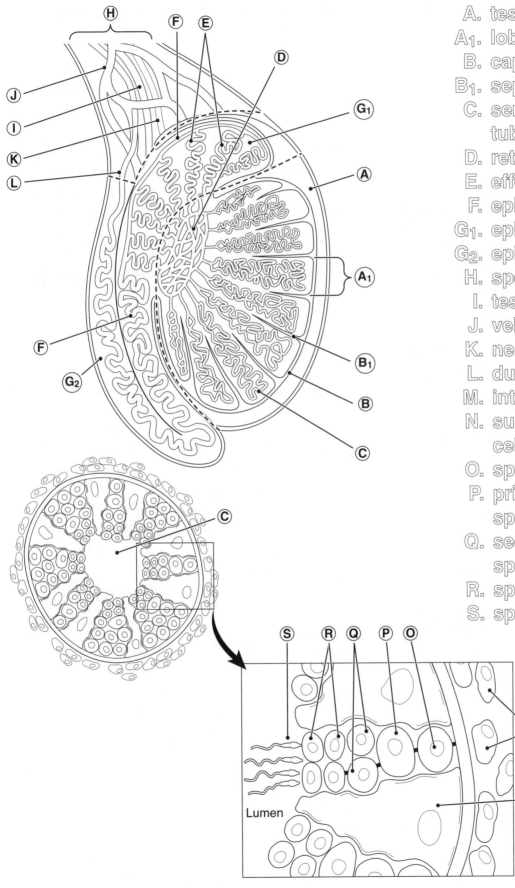

A. testis
A₁. lobule
B. capsule
B₁. septum
C. seminiferous
   tubule
D. rete testis
E. efferent duct
F. epididymal duct
G₁. epididymis head
G₂. epididymis body
H. spermatic cord
I. testicular artery
J. veins
K. nerves
L. ductus deferens
M. interstitial cells
N. sustentacular
   cell
O. spermatogonium
P. primary
   spermatocyte
Q. secondary
   spermatocyte
R. spermatids
S. spermatozoon

Lumen

Coloring Exercise 13-3 ➤ The Female Reproductive System

Anatomy of the Female Reproductive System

The top figure at right shows a sagittal view; see Coloring Exercise 13-4 for a frontal view.

	Structure	Function
Mons pubis Ⓐ	Adipose tissue covered by skin and hair	Protects **pubic symphysis** Ⓑ
Labia	Inner (**labium minus** Ⓒ) and outer (**labium majus** Ⓓ)	Protection
Clitoris Ⓔ	Erectile tissue	Sexual excitement
Vagina Ⓕ	Muscular blind-ended tube; the **posterior fornix** (F1) may be partially covered by **hymen** Ⓖ; anterior to **rectum** Ⓗ and posterior to **bladder** Ⓘ and **urethra** Ⓙ	Sexual intercourse, passage of menstrual flow, childbirth
Uterus Ⓚ (see Coloring Exercise 13-4)	Muscular pear-shaped organ supported by **round ligament** Ⓛ and **uterosacral ligament** Ⓜ	Nurtures and houses fetus
Cervix Ⓝ	Neck of uterus; contains cervical canal	Passage of menstrual flow and spermatozoa; passage of baby from uterus to vagina
Ovaries Ⓞ (see Coloring Exercise 13-4)	Oval bodies consisting of follicles (gametes) and connective tissue	Generate ova (eggs) and hormones (estrogen, progesterone)
Oviducts Ⓟ	Small muscular tubes	Convey ovum to uterus, sperm to meet ovum
Obstetrical perineum Ⓠ	Pelvic floor area between **anus** Ⓡ and **vagina** Ⓕ	

✎ **COLORING INSTRUCTIONS**

1. Color both figures at the same time.
2. Use the same color for the vagina Ⓕ and the posterior fornix (F1).
3. Use dark colors for the clitoris Ⓔ and the urethra/urethral opening Ⓙ, because these structures are small.
4. Use related colors for the uterus Ⓚ and the cervix Ⓝ.

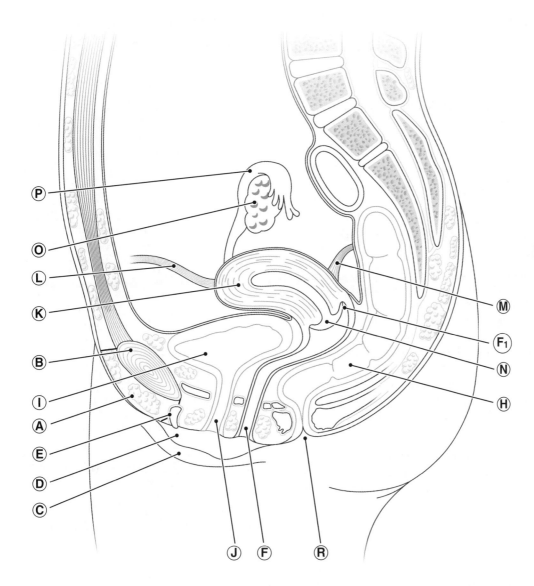

A. mons pubis
B. pubic symphysis
C. labium minus
D. labium majus
E. clitoris
F. vagina
F₁. posterior fornix
G. hymen
H. rectum
I. bladder
J. urethra
K. uterus
L. round ligament
M. uterosacral ligament
N. cervix
O. ovaries
P. oviducts
Q. obstetrical perineum
R. anus

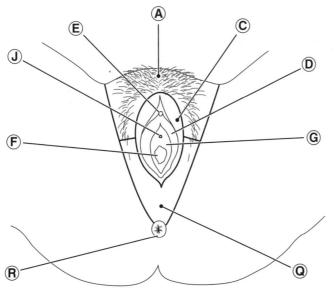

Coloring Exercise 13-4 ➤ Fertilization: Spermatozoa and the Female Internal Reproductive Organs

Female Reproductive System: Anatomy (2)

The top figure highlights aspects of female reproductive anatomy not visible in Coloring Exercise 13-3.

- **Broad ligament** (A) supports the internal reproductive organs and anchors them to the abdominal wall
- **Vagina** (B)
  - Contains numerous folds (**rugae** (B1))
  - Greater **vestibular glands** (C) secrete mucus into vagina
- Uterus
  - Three anatomic divisions:
    - **Fundus** (D): dome-shaped portion above oviducts
    - **Body** (E): most muscular part of uterus
    - **Cervix** (F): narrowest part, contains cervical canal
  - Uterine wall has three layers:
    - Inner **endometrium** (G): blood vessels, glands
    - Middle **myometrium** (H): smooth muscle
    - Outer **perimetrium** (I): connective tissue
- **Oviduct** (J) has fingerlike extensions (**fimbriae** (J1)) that envelop ovary, pick up ovum
- **Ovary** (K)
  - Joined to the uterus by the **ovarian ligament** (L)
  - Consists of connective tissue and FOLLICLES
  - Each follicle contains an egg (ovum); released during ovulation (see below and Coloring Exercise 13-5)

Events in Fertilization

- **Spermatozoa** (N) (see below) travel through vagina, uterus, and oviduct
- **Ovum** (M) released from **ovary** (K), picked up by **fimbriae** (J1), travels a short distance through the **oviduct** (J)
- One spermatozoon penetrates outer surface of ovum; sperm head enters ovum
- Fertilized ovum (**zygote** (O)) travels to uterus (developing as it goes), embeds in **endometrium** (G) as a **blastocyst** (O)

Structure of a Spermatozoon (N)

- **Head** (P)
  - **Nucleus** (Q): contains 23 chromosomes
  - **Acrosome** (R): enzyme-containing cap
    - Releases enzymes when sperm meets egg
    - Helps sperm penetrate egg covering
- **Midpiece** (S): contains **mitochondria** (T)
  - Generates energy for swimming
- **Tail** (U): contains **flagellum** (V)
  - Propels sperm through female reproductive tract

🖊 **COLORING INSTRUCTIONS**

Color each structure and its name at the same time, using the same color. Read all instructions before you start. On the top figure:

1. Color parts (A) to (L), but use very light shading for the vagina (B) and oviducts (J). Use the same color scheme as in the previous exercise.

2. LIGHTLY SHADE the anatomic divisions of the uterus (D) to (F), as indicated by the dotted lines. Do not color the cross-section portions.

3. Color the layers of the uterine wall (G) to (I) in cross-section only.

🖊 **COLORING INSTRUCTIONS**

On the top figure:

1. Trace the arrows representing the voyage of sperm (N) towards the ovum (M).

2. Color the ovum and the arrows representing the pathway of the ovum.

3. Color the cartoon of fertilization (far right).

4. Color the arrows representing the pathway of the zygote (O) to its implantation site.

🖊 **COLORING INSTRUCTIONS**

On the bottom figure:

1. Lightly shade the three portions of the spermatozoon (P), (S), (U), which are divided by dotted lines.

2. Color the internal structures (Q), (R), (T), (V). Note that the acrosome overlies the nucleus.

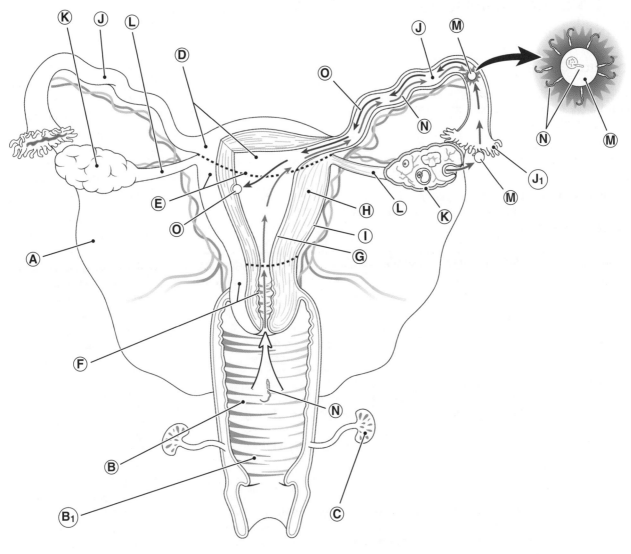

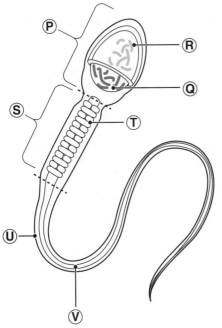

A. broad ligament
B. vagina
B₁. rugae
C. vestibular glands
D. fundus
E. body
F. cervix
G. endometrium
H. myometrium
I. perimetrium
J. oviduct
J₁. fimbrae
K. ovary

L. ovarian
   ligament
M. ovum
N. spermatozoa
O. zygote
   blastocyst
P. head
Q. nucleus
R. acrosome
S. midpiece
T. mitochondria
U. tail
V. flagellum

Coloring Exercise 13-5 ➤ The Menstrual Cycle

Menstrual Cycle

- Cyclic changes in the pituitary gland, ovary, and uterus that produce a gamete (**ovum** Ⓐ), encourage fertilization of the ovum, and prepare the body to nourish the fertilized ovum
- Average duration 22-45 days
  - Day 1: first day of menstrual bleeding
- Divided into three phases:
  - **Follicular phase** Ⓑ: before ovulation
  - **Ovulation** Ⓒ: release of the egg from the ovary
  - **Luteal phase** Ⓓ: after ovulation

	Follicular Phase Ⓑ	Ovulation Ⓒ	Luteal Phase Ⓓ
Pituitary Hormones	**FSH** Ⓔ secretion decreases; **LH** Ⓕ levels remain low	**LH** levels Ⓕ (and secondarily **FSH** levels Ⓔ) dramatically increase (LH surge)	**FSH** Ⓔ and **LH** Ⓕ levels rapidly decrease; levels increase when corpus luteum regresses
Ovarian Events	FSH stimulates development of **immature follicle** Ⓖ into **mature follicle** Ⓗ	LH stimulates ovulation: **ovulating follicle** Ⓘ releases **ovum** Ⓐ into peritoneal space	LH stimulates conversion of **ovulating follicle** Ⓘ into **corpus luteum** Ⓙ; corpus luteum eventually regresses if ovum is not fertilized
Ovarian Hormones	**Estrogen** Ⓚ secretion increases in parallel with follicular size; estrogen inhibits FSH secretion	**Estrogen** Ⓚ levels begin to fall; **progesterone** Ⓛ levels begin to rise	**Estrogen** Ⓚ and **progesterone** Ⓛ secretion varies in accordance with corpus luteum size
Uterine Cycle	**Menstruation** Ⓜ: **endometrium** Ⓝ sloughed off in **menstrual flow** Ⓞ due to low estrogen and progesterone; **Proliferative phase** Ⓟ: rising estrogen levels stimulate endometrial proliferation		**Secretory phase** Ⓠ: estrogen stimulates endometrial proliferation, progesterone stimulates **glycogen secretion** Ⓡ

✎ COLORING INSTRUCTIONS

Color each figure part and its name at the same time, using the same color.

1. LIGHTLY shade the left Ⓑ and right Ⓓ portions of the entire diagram, representing the follicular and luteal phases (respectively). Note there is a small area of Ⓑ on the far right of the diagram.

2. Use a dark, bright color to outline the line representing ovulation Ⓒ.

3. Color the areas of the graph representing changes in FSH Ⓔ and LH Ⓕ levels.

4. Color the figures representing the different stages of development of the follicle and corpus luteum (Ⓖ to Ⓙ). Use a contrasting color for the ovum Ⓐ within each follicle. Color these elements on bottom figure as well.

5. Color the areas of the graph representing changes in estrogen Ⓚ and progesterone Ⓛ levels and the arrows.

6. Color the bars underneath the diagram, representing the phases of the uterine cycle (Ⓜ, Ⓟ, Ⓠ).

7. Lightly color the endometrium Ⓝ as it changes throughout the cycle.

8. Color the glycogen-rich secretion Ⓡ of the secretory phase and the menstrual discharge Ⓞ of the menstrual phase.

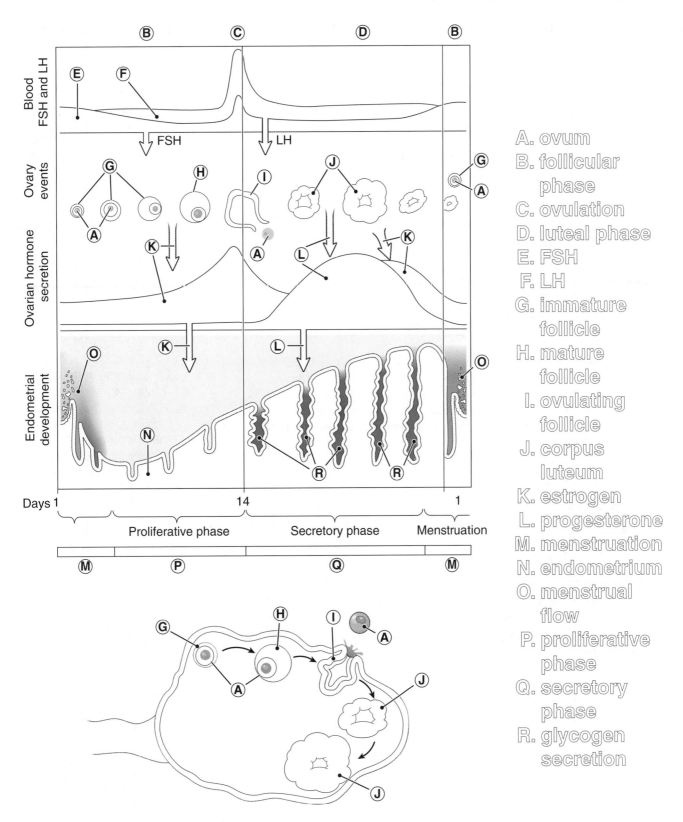

A. ovum
B. follicular
   phase
C. ovulation
D. luteal phase
E. FSH
F. LH
G. immature
   follicle
H. mature
   follicle
I. ovulating
   follicle
J. corpus
   luteum
K. estrogen
L. progesterone
M. menstruation
N. endometrium
O. menstrual
   flow
P. proliferative
   phase
Q. secretory
   phase
R. glycogen
   secretion

Coloring Exercise 13-6 ➤ The Placenta and Fetal Circulation

The Placenta

- Organ unique to pregnancy
- Secretes hormones to maintain the pregnancy (progesterone, estrogen, human chorionic gonadotropin)
- Exchanges nutrients and wastes between mother and fetus, but does not allow fetal and maternal blood to mix

Structure of the Placenta

- Maternal Portion
  - Derived from uterus endometrium
  - **Uterine arterioles** Ⓐ deliver oxygen-rich blood
  - **Venous sinus** Ⓑ is a pool of oxygen-rich blood
  - **Uterine veins** Ⓒ drain away oxygen-poor blood
- Fetal Portion
  - Two **umbilical arteries** Ⓓ deliver mixed blood from the fetus
  - Umbilical capillaries exchange substances with the venous sinus
    - Oxygen and nutrients diffuse from sinus to capillaries
    - Carbon dioxide and waste products diffuse from capillaries to sinus
    - **Mixed blood enters capillary** Ⓔ; **oxygen-rich blood leaves capillary** Ⓕ
  - **Umbilical vein** Ⓖ returns oxygen-rich blood to fetus

The Fetal Circulation

- **Umbilical vein** Ⓖ delivers oxygen-rich blood from placenta
- Some blood delivered to cells of **liver** Ⓗ; most blood bypasses liver, passing through **ductus venosus** Ⓘ
- Blood joins **oxygen-poor blood** from lower **inferior vena cava** Ⓙ
- **Mixed blood** in the upper **inferior vena cava** Ⓚ enters **heart** Ⓛ
- Blood in heart can take multiple paths to bypass lungs
  - Some passes through **foramen ovale** Ⓜ into left heart and **aorta** Ⓝ
  - Some enters **pulmonary vessels** Ⓞ but diverted into aorta via the **ductus arteriosus** Ⓟ
  - Very little passes through entire pulmonary circulation into left heart and aorta
- Mixed blood transported by **aorta** Ⓝ to fetal tissues
  - Fetal hemoglobin is very efficient; fetus receives adequate oxygen from mixed blood
- **Umbilical arteries** Ⓓ branch off from **internal iliac arteries** Ⓠ; return blood to placenta

---

✍ COLORING INSTRUCTIONS

Color each figure part and its name at the same time, using the same color. Read these general instructions before proceeding:

1. Use variants of red for vessels containing oxygen-rich blood (Ⓐ, Ⓑ, Ⓕ, and Ⓘ) and variants of blue for vessels containing oxygen-poor blood (Ⓒ and Ⓙ).
2. Use variants of purple for all other vessels, since they contain mixed blood.

✍ COLORING INSTRUCTIONS

On the bottom left figure:

1. Color the uterine arterioles Ⓐ red and the uterine venules Ⓒ blue.
2. Color the venous sinus Ⓑ red and the two umbilical arteries Ⓓ arriving at the placenta purple.
3. Color the arterial end of the placental capillaries Ⓕ purple, and the venous end red Ⓔ. Color the umbilical vein and its branches Ⓖ purple as well.

✍ COLORING INSTRUCTIONS

On the main figure:

1. Starting from the placental side, color the rest of the umbilical vein Ⓖ.
2. LIGHTLY shade the liver Ⓗ, and color the ductus venosus Ⓘ red.
3. Color the lower portion of the inferior vena cava Ⓙ blue and the upper portion Ⓚ purple.
5. Use variants of purple to color structures Ⓛ, Ⓞ, Ⓝ, Ⓠ, and Ⓓ.
6. Use bright colors for the foramen ovale Ⓜ (a small circle) and the ductus arteriosus Ⓟ (a short vessel).

A. uterine arterioles
B. venous sinus
C. uterine veins
D. umbilical arteries
E. umbilical capillaries
   (mixed)
F. umbilical capillaries
   (high O₂)
G. umbilical vein
H. liver
 I. ductus venous
J. inferior vena
   cava (low O₂)
K. inverior vena
   cava (mixed)

☐ Oxygen-rich blood
☐ Oxygen-poor blood
☐ Mixed blood

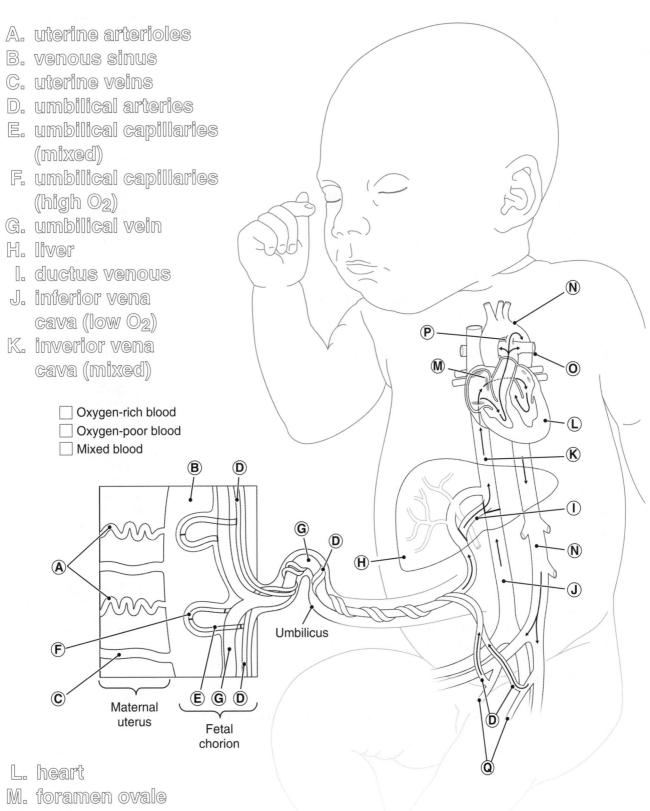

Umbilicus

Maternal
uterus

Fetal
chorion

L. heart
M. foramen ovale
N. aorta
O. pulmonary vessels
P. ductus arteriosus
Q. internal iliac arteries

Coloring Exercise 13-7 ➤ Mammary Glands and Lactation

Mammary Glands

- Part of reproductive system (accessory organs)
- Modified sweat glands

Structure

- Overlie **pectoralis major** Ⓐ muscle and **ribs** Ⓑ
- Mostly composed of **adipose tissue** Ⓒ (fat), especially in women not producing milk
- Tissue supported by numerous **suspensory ligaments** Ⓓ
- Glandular (milk-producing) tissue organized in **lobules** Ⓔ
- Each lobule drains into **lactiferous duct** Ⓕ
- Lactiferous ducts have dilated region, **lactiferous sinus** Ⓖ
  - Milk stored in ducts and sinuses
- Lactiferous ducts terminate in small holes in the **nipple** Ⓗ
- Nipple surrounded by a pigmented area, the **areola** Ⓘ

Development

- Enlarge during puberty
  - Estrogen stimulates fat deposition, duct development
  - Progesterone stimulates gland development
- Become functional late in pregnancy
  - Placental lactogen (prolactin-like hormone) secreted by the placenta stimulates further breast development
- Become active after childbirth
  - First secretion: colostrum
    - High in sugar, antibodies
  - After a few days: breasts secrete milk

Regulation

- **Baby** Ⓛ suckling at breast activates **sensory pathways** Ⓜ, which eventually activate neurons in the **hypothalamus** Ⓝ
  - Sight, smell, sound, or thought of a baby can also activate these pathways
- Hypothalamus stimulates the secretion of **prolactin** Ⓙ from the **anterior pituitary gland** Ⓞ
  - Prolactin stimulates milk synthesis by the **lobules** Ⓔ
- Hypothalamus produces **oxytocin** Ⓚ; released from the **posterior pituitary gland** Ⓟ
  - Oxytocin stimulates contraction of **milk ducts** Ⓕ—milk is ejected from the **nipple** Ⓗ

🖎 **COLORING INSTRUCTIONS**

Color each structure and its name at the same time, using the same color. On the left-hand figure:

1. Color the structures found in the breast (Ⓐ to Ⓘ). This figure shows the breast of a woman actively producing milk.

2. Use related colors for the lactiferous ducts Ⓕ and the lactiferous sinuses Ⓖ.

🖎 **COLORING INSTRUCTIONS**

On the right-hand figure:

1. Color the suckling baby Ⓛ, the arrow representing the sensory pathway Ⓜ, and the hypothalamus Ⓝ.

2. Color the anterior pituitary gland Ⓞ, the arrow representing prolactin action Ⓙ, and the lobules Ⓔ. Use related colors for these structures.

3. Color the posterior pituitary gland Ⓟ, the arrow representing oxytocin action Ⓚ, and the ducts Ⓕ. Use related colors for these structures.

4. Color the nipple Ⓗ.

A. pectoralis major
B. rib
C. adipose tissue
D. suspensory
   ligament
E. lobule
F. lactiferous ducts
G. lactiferous sinus
H. nipple
I. areola
J. prolactin
K. oxytocin
L. baby
M. sensory pathway
N. hypothalamus
O. anterior pituitary
   gland
P. posterior pituitary
   gland

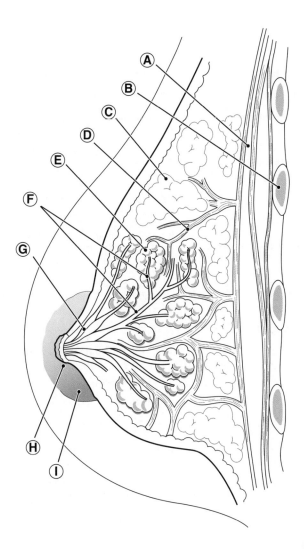

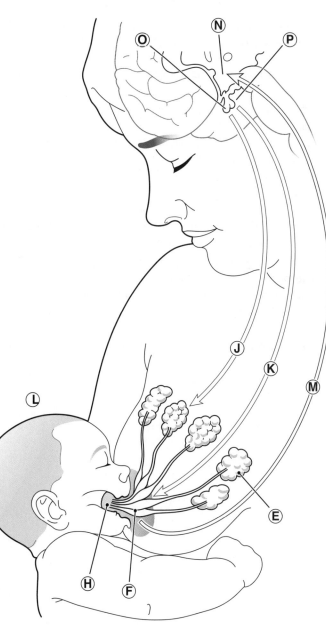

Coloring Exercise 13-8 ➤ Meiosis and Heredity

Meiosis

- **Meiosis** Ⓐ generates gametes: **spermatozoa** Ⓑ and **ova** Ⓒ
- Human cells contain 46 chromosomes, organized in 23 pairs
- Each pair includes one maternal (from **mother** Ⓓ) and one paternal (from **father** Ⓔ) chromosome
- One pair (sex chromosomes) determines gender
  - Mother = two **X chromosomes** Ⓕ
  - Father = one X chromosome, one **Y chromosome** Ⓖ
- **Meiosis** Ⓐ generates gametes with 23 chromosomes, one from each pair
  - Zygote formed by the union of the two gametes; zygote will have 46 chromosomes

Sex Chromosomes and Meiosis

- The figure at right traces the sex chromosomes through the generation of spermatozoa (spermatogenesis) and ova (oogenesis) and their union into a new individual
  - Spermatogenesis also illustrated in Coloring Exercise 13-2
  - Figure does not show the other 22 chromosome pairs
- Paternal **spermatogonium** Ⓗ (sperm stem cell) contains 1 **X chromosome** Ⓕ and 1 **Y chromosome** Ⓖ
  - Meiosis divides the chromosome pair
    - Half of the **spermatozoa** Ⓑ receive an **X chromosome** Ⓕ
    - Half receive a **Y chromosome** Ⓖ
- Maternal **oogonium** Ⓘ (ovum stem cell) contains 2 **X chromosomes** Ⓕ
  - **Meiosis** divides the chromosome pair
    - All **ova** Ⓒ receive an **X chromosome** Ⓕ
- Offspring gender depends on sperm cell's sex chromosome
  - **Male baby** Ⓔ₁: results from Y chromosome sperm
  - **Female baby** Ⓓ₁: results from X chromosome sperm

COLORING INSTRUCTIONS

Color each figure part and its name at the same time, using the same color. On the top figure:

1. Use variants of blue to color the father Ⓔ, and lightly shade the spermatogonium Ⓗ and the spermatozoon Ⓑ.
2. Color the arrow representing meiosis Ⓐ.
3. Color the larger, X chromosome Ⓕ and the smaller Y chromosome Ⓖ in the spermatogonium and sperm, using contrasting colors.
4. Use variants of red to color the mother Ⓓ and lightly shade the oogonium Ⓘ and ovum Ⓒ.
5. Color the X chromosomes Ⓕ in the oogonium and ovum.

COLORING INSTRUCTIONS

On the bottom figure:

1. Lightly shade the ova Ⓒ and sperm Ⓑ.
2. Color the X Ⓕ and Y Ⓖ chromosomes in the gametes.
3. Lightly shade the male babies (and the fertilized eggs that produce them) Ⓔ₁, using a variant of blue, then color the chromosomes.
4. Repeat step 3 for the female babies Ⓓ₁, using a variant of red.

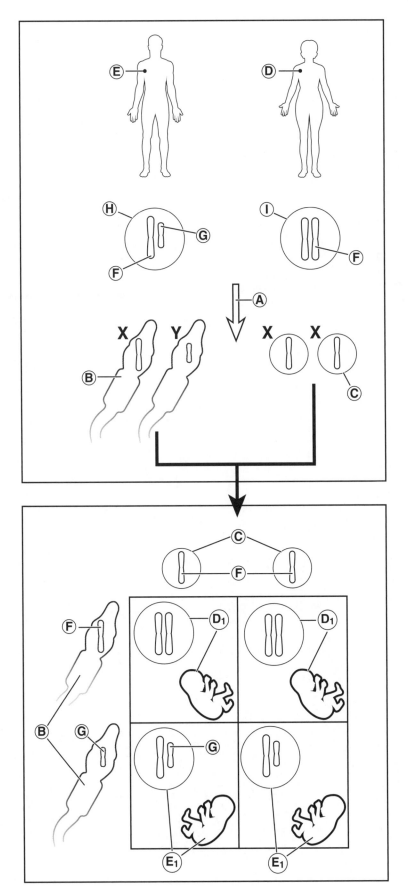

A. meiosis
B. spermatozoon
C. ovum
D. mother
D_1. female baby
E. father
E_1. male baby
F. X chromosome
G. Y chromosome
H. spermatogonium
I. oogonium

Appendix I ➤ Answers to Coloring Exercises 3-1, 4-10, and 4-11

Coloring Exercise 3-1

A. cranium
B. facial bones
C. mandible
D. sternum
E. costal cartilage
F. ribs
G. vertebral column
H. sacrum
I. clavicle
J. scapula
K. humerus
L. radius
M. ulna
N. carpals
O. metacarpals
P. phalanges
Q. ilium (of pelvis)
R. pelvis
S. femur
T. patella
U. fibula
V. tibia
W. tarsals
X. phalanges
Y. metatarsals
Z. calcaneus

Coloring Exercise 4-10

A. temporalis
B. obicularis oculi
C. obicularis oris
D. masseter
E. sternocleidomastoid
F. trapezius
G. deltoid
H. pectoralis major
I. serratus anterior

J. intercostals
K. external oblique
L. internal oblique
M. rectus abdominis
N. abdominal aponeurosis
O. biceps brachii
P. brachioradialis
Q. flexor carpi
R. extensor carpi
S. adductors of thigh
T. sartorius
U. quadriceps femoris
V. gastrocnemius
W. soleus
X. peroneus longus
Y. tibialis anterior

Coloring Exercise 4-11

A. sternocleidomastoid
B. trapezius
C. deltoid
D. teres minor
E. teres major
F. latissimus dorsi
G. triceps brachii
H. gluteus maximus
I. biceps femoris
J. semitendinosus
K. semimembranosus
L. gastrocnemius
M. peroneus longus
N. lumbodorsal fascia
O. iliotibial tract
P. olecranon
Q. Achilles tendon
R. gluteus medius
S. epicranial aponeurosis
T. hamstring group

Appendix II > Pull-Out and Color Flashcards

The flashcards on the following pages zoom in on some figures from the coloring exercises in the chapters. Pull these out and color them alongside the matching coloring exercises, then use them for portable study and review. If you like, you can color the circle next to the term with the color you used for the figure part.

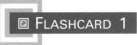
Coloring Exercise 3-6

- Ⓐ mandible ◯
- Ⓑ maxillae ◯
- Ⓒ zygomatic bone ◯
- Ⓓ nasal bone ◯
- Ⓔ lacrimal bone ◯
- Ⓕ vomer ◯
- Ⓗ inferior nasal conchae ◯
- Ⓘ frontal bone ◯
- Ⓙ parietal bone ◯
- Ⓞ temporal bone ◯
- Ⓠ ethmoid bone ◯
- Ⓡ sphenoid bone ◯

Coloring Exercise 3-6

- Ⓓ nasal bone ◯
- Ⓔ lacrimal bone ◯
- Ⓘ frontal bone ◯
- Ⓙ parietal bone ◯
- Ⓚ coronal suture ◯
- Ⓛ squamous suture ◯
- Ⓝ sagittal suture ◯
- Ⓟ occipital bone ◯
- Ⓡ sphenoid bone ◯

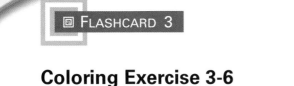
Coloring Exercise 3-6

- Ⓐ mandible ◯
- Ⓑ maxillae ◯
- Ⓒ zygomatic bone ◯
- Ⓜ lambdoid suture ◯
- Ⓞ temporal bone ◯
- Ⓞ₁ styloid process ◯
- Ⓞ₂ mastoid process ◯
- Ⓞ₃ zygomatic process ◯
- Ⓢ hyoid bone ◯

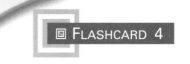
Coloring Exercise 3-7

- Ⓐ cervical vertebrae ◯
- Ⓑ atlas ◯
- Ⓒ axis ◯
- Ⓓ thoracic vertebrae ◯
- Ⓔ lumbar vertebrae ◯
- Ⓕ sacrum ◯
- Ⓖ coccyx ◯
- Ⓗ intervertebral disc ◯
- Ⓘ body ◯
- Ⓚ intervertebral foramen ◯
- Ⓛ spinous process ◯
- Ⓜ transverse process ◯

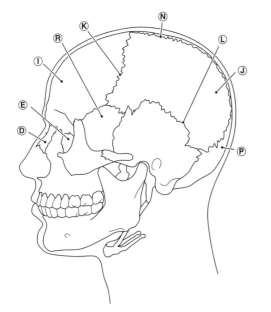

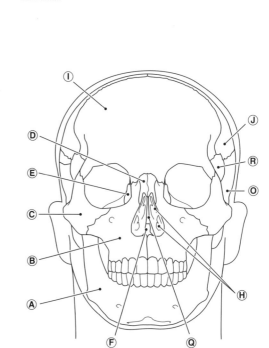

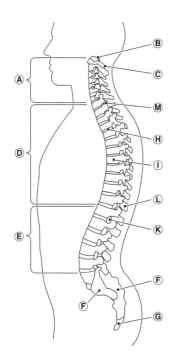

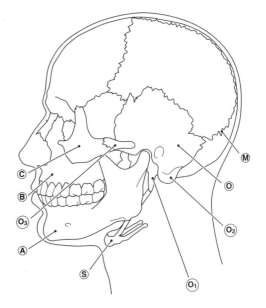

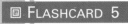

FLASHCARD 5

Coloring Exercise 3-8

- Ⓐ sternum ○
- Ⓐ₁ manubrium ○
- Ⓐ₂ clavicular notch ○
- Ⓐ₃ body ○
- Ⓐ₄ sternal notch ○
- Ⓐ₅ xiphoid process ○
- Ⓑ costal cartilage ○
- Ⓒ true ribs ○
- Ⓓ false ribs ○
- Ⓔ false (floating) ribs ○
- Ⓕ intercostal space ○

FLASHCARD 6

Coloring Exercise 3-8

- Ⓖ clavicle ○
- Ⓗ scapula ○
- Ⓗ₁ spine ○
- Ⓗ₂ supraspinous fossa ○
- Ⓗ₃ infraspinous fossa ○
- Ⓗ₄ coracoid process ○
- Ⓗ₅ acromion ○
- Ⓗ₆ glenoid cavity ○
- Ⓘ humerus ○

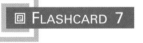

FLASHCARD 7

Coloring Exercise 3-9

- Ⓐ humerus ○
- Ⓐ₁ head ○
- Ⓐ₂ medial epicondyle ○
- Ⓐ₃ lateral epicondyle ○
- Ⓐ₄ trochlea ○
- Ⓐ₅ capitulum ○
- Ⓐ₆ radial fossa ○
- Ⓐ₇ olecranon fossa ○

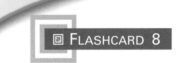

FLASHCARD 8

Coloring Exercise 3-9

- Ⓑ ulna ○
- Ⓑ₁ head ○
- Ⓑ₂ olecranon ○
- Ⓑ₃ trochlear notch ○
- Ⓑ₄ radial notch ○
- Ⓑ₅ styloid process ○
- Ⓒ radius ○
- Ⓒ₁ head ○
- Ⓒ₂ neck ○
- Ⓒ₃ styloid process ○

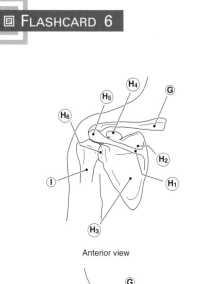

Anterior view

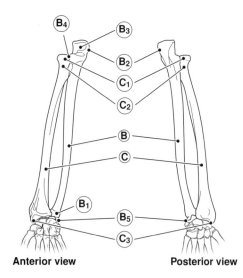

Posterior view

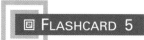

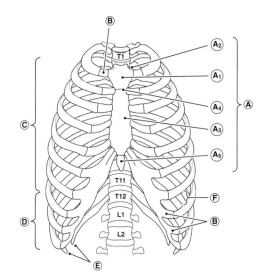

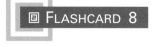

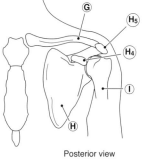

Anterior view   **Posterior view**

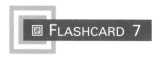

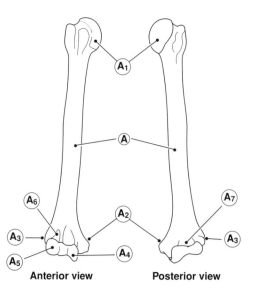

Anterior view   **Posterior view**

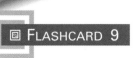

Coloring Exercise 3-10

- Ⓐ ilium ○
- Ⓐ₁ iliac crest ○
- Ⓐ₂ anterior superior iliac spine ○
- Ⓑ ischium ○
- Ⓑ₁ ischial tuberosity ○
- Ⓑ₂ ischial spine ○
- Ⓒ pubis ○
- Ⓓ acetabulum ○
- Ⓔ sacrum ○
- Ⓕ pubic symphysis ○
- Ⓖ pubic arch ○
- Ⓗ obdurator foramen ○

▣ FLASHCARD 10

Coloring Exercise 3-11

- Ⓐ femur ○
- Ⓐ₁ head ○
- Ⓐ₂ neck ○
- Ⓐ₃ greater trochanter ○
- Ⓐ₄ lesser trochanter ○
- Ⓐ₅ linea aspera ○
- Ⓐ₆ medial condyle ○
- Ⓐ₇ lateral condyle ○
- Ⓐ₈ patellar surface ○
- Ⓐ₉ medial epicondyle ○

▣ FLASHCARD 11

Coloring Exercise 3-11

- Ⓓ tibia ○
- Ⓓ₁ lateral condyle ○
- Ⓓ₂ medial condyle ○
- Ⓓ₃ anterior crest ○
- Ⓓ₄ medial malleolus ○
- Ⓔ fibula ○
- Ⓔ₁ head ○
- Ⓔ₂ lateral malleolus ○

▣ FLASHCARD 12

Coloring Exercise 3-12

- Ⓐ scaphoid ○
- Ⓑ lunate ○
- Ⓒ triquetral ○
- Ⓓ pisiform ○
- Ⓔ trapezium ○
- Ⓕ trapezoid ○
- Ⓖ capitate ○
- Ⓗ hamate ○
- Ⓝ metacarpals ○
- Ⓟ proximal phalanx ○
- Ⓠ middle phalanx ○
- Ⓡ distal phalanx ○
- Ⓤ radius ○
- Ⓥ ulna ○

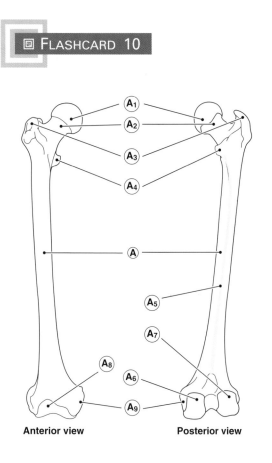

A₁
A₂
A₃
A₄
A
A₅
A₇
A₈
A₆
A₉

Anterior view   **Posterior view**

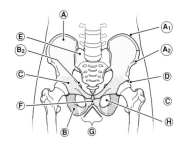

A
E
B₂
C
F
B
G
A₁
A₂
D
C
H

Anterior view

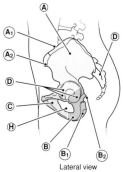

A
A₁
A₂
D
D
C
H
B
B₁
B₂

Lateral view

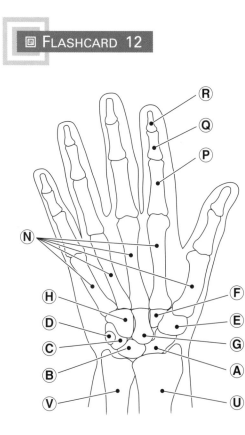

R
Q
P
N
H
D
C
B
V
F
E
G
A
U

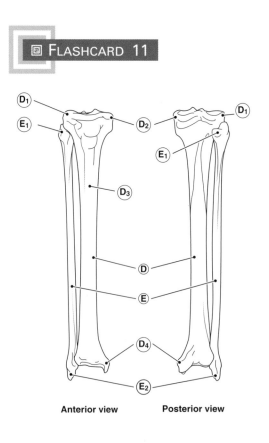

D₁
E₁
D₂
D₁
E₁
D₃
D
E
D₄
E₂

Anterior view   **Posterior view**

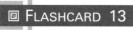

Coloring Exercise 3-12

Ⓘ cuboid ◯
Ⓙ cuneiforms ◯
Ⓚ navicular ◯
Ⓛ talus ◯
Ⓜ calcaneus ◯
Ⓞ metatarsals ◯
Ⓟ proximal phalanx ◯
Ⓠ middle phalanx ◯
Ⓡ distal phalanx ◯
Ⓢ fibula ◯
Ⓣ tibia ◯

Coloring Exercise 4-6

Ⓐ frontalis ◯
Ⓑ obicularis oris ◯
Ⓒ nasalis ◯
Ⓓ quadratus labii superioris ◯
Ⓔ zygomaticus ◯
Ⓕ obicularis oris ◯
Ⓖ quadratus labii superioris ◯
Ⓗ mentalis ◯
Ⓘ triangularis ◯
Ⓙ buccinator ◯
Ⓚ digastricus ◯
Ⓛ masseter ◯
Ⓜ sternocleidomastoid ◯
Ⓝ temporalis ◯
Ⓞ trapezius ◯

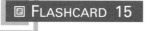

Coloring Exercise 4-6

Ⓐ frontalis ◯
Ⓑ obicularis oris ◯
Ⓒ nasalis ◯
Ⓓ quadratus labii superioris ◯
Ⓔ zygomaticus ◯
Ⓕ obicularis oris ◯
Ⓗ mentalis ◯
Ⓘ triangularis ◯
Ⓛ masseter ◯
Ⓜ sternocleidomastoid ◯
Ⓝ temporalis ◯

Coloring Exercise 4-8

Ⓐ trapezius ◯
Ⓑ latissimus dorsi ◯
Ⓒ pectoralis major ◯
Ⓓ serratus anterior ◯
Ⓖ deltoid ◯
Ⓗ biceps brachii ◯
Ⓘ brachioradialis ◯
Ⓚ brachialis ◯
Ⓜ flexor carpi radialis ◯
Ⓝ flexor carpi ulnaris ◯
Ⓟ flexor digitorum superficialis ◯

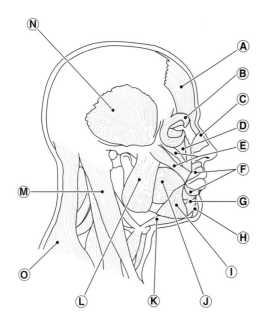

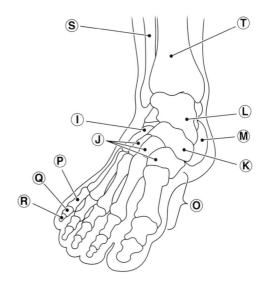

Anterior view

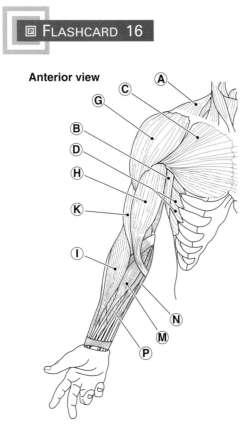

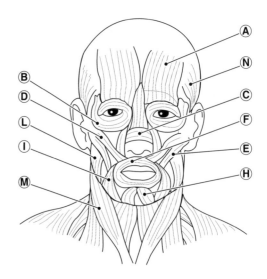

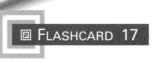

Coloring Exercise 4-8

- Ⓐ trapezius ○
- Ⓑ latissimus dorsi ○
- Ⓔ teres major ○
- Ⓕ teres minor ○
- Ⓖ deltoid ○
- Ⓙ triceps brachii ○
- Ⓛ extensor carpi radialis longus ○
- Ⓝ flexor carpi ulnaris ○
- Ⓞ extensor carpi ulnaris ○
- Ⓠ extensor digitorum ○
- Ⓡ lumbodorsal fascia ○

Coloring Exercise 4-9

- Ⓐ iliopsoas ○
- Ⓑ sartorius ○
- Ⓒ rectus femoris ○
- Ⓓ vastus lateralis ○
- Ⓔ vastus medialis ○
- Ⓕ adductor longus ○
- Ⓖ gracilis ○
- Ⓗ adductor magnus ○
- Ⓣ iliotibial tract ○

Coloring Exercise 4-9

- Ⓑ sartorius ○
- Ⓖ gracilis ○
- Ⓗ adductor magnus ○
- Ⓘ gluteus medius ○
- Ⓙ gluteus maximus ○
- Ⓚ biceps femoris ○
- Ⓛ semitendinosus ○
- Ⓜ semimembranosus ○
- Ⓣ iliotibial tract ○

Coloring Exercise 4-9

- Ⓝ peroneus longus ○
- Ⓞ tibialis anterior ○
- Ⓟ gastrocnemius ○
- Ⓠ soleus ○
- Ⓡ extensor digitorum longus ○
- Ⓢ flexor digitorum longus ○

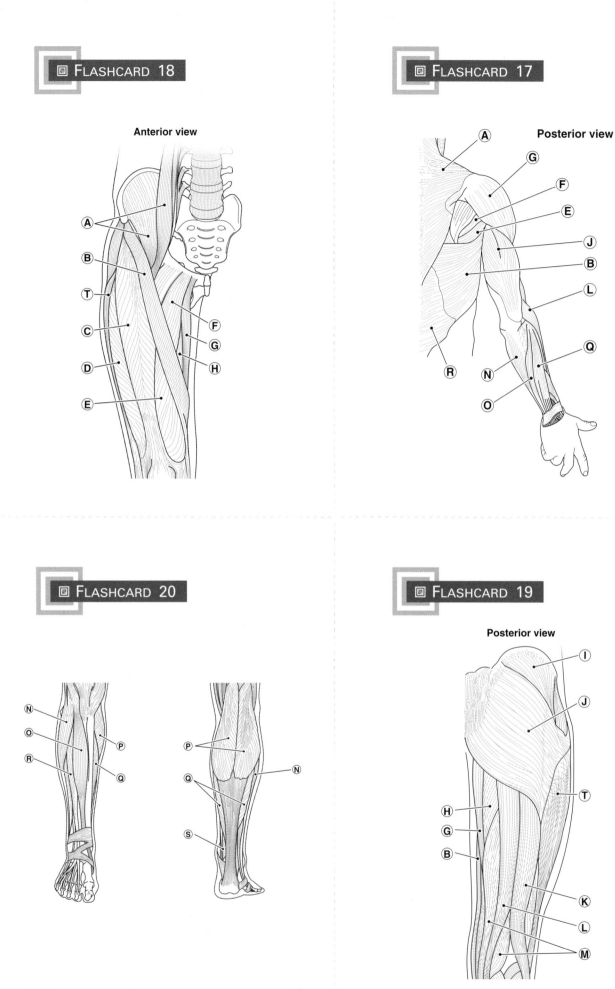

Anterior view

Posterior view

Posterior view

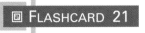

FLASHCARD 21

Coloring Exercise 4-10

- Ⓔ sternocleidomastoid ◯
- Ⓕ trapezius ◯
- Ⓘ serratus anterior ◯
- Ⓙ intercostals ◯
- Ⓚ external obliques ◯
- Ⓛ internal obliques ◯
- Ⓜ rectus abdominus ◯
- Ⓝ abdominal aponeurosis ◯

FLASHCARD 22

Coloring Exercise 5-7

- Ⓐ cerebrum ◯
- Ⓑ corpus callosum ◯
- Ⓕ hypothalamus ◯
- Ⓖ pituitary gland ◯
- Ⓗ thalamus ◯
- ⑪ cerebellar cortex ◯
- ⑫ cerebellar medulla ◯
- Ⓙ midbrain ◯
- Ⓚ pons ◯
- Ⓛ medulla oblongata ◯
- Ⓜ spinal cord ◯

FLASHCARD 23

Coloring Exercise 5-7

- Ⓐⁱ cerebral cortex ◯
- Ⓐ² cerebral white matter ◯
- Ⓑ corpus callosum ◯
- Ⓒ caudate nucleus ◯
- Ⓓ putamen ◯
- Ⓔ globus pallidus ◯
- Ⓕ hypothalamus ◯
- Ⓗ thalamus ◯

FLASHCARD 24

Coloring Exercise 5-8

- Ⓐ central sulcus ◯
- Ⓑ lateral sulcus ◯
- Ⓒ frontal lobe ◯
- Ⓓ primary motor area ◯
- Ⓔ¹ written speech area ◯
- Ⓔ² motor speech area ◯
- Ⓕ parietal lobe ◯
- Ⓖ primary sensory area ◯
- Ⓗ temporal lobe ◯
- ⑪ auditory receiving area ◯
- ⑫ auditory association area ◯
- ⑬ Wernicke area ◯
- Ⓙ occipital lobe ◯
- Ⓚ visual receiving area ◯

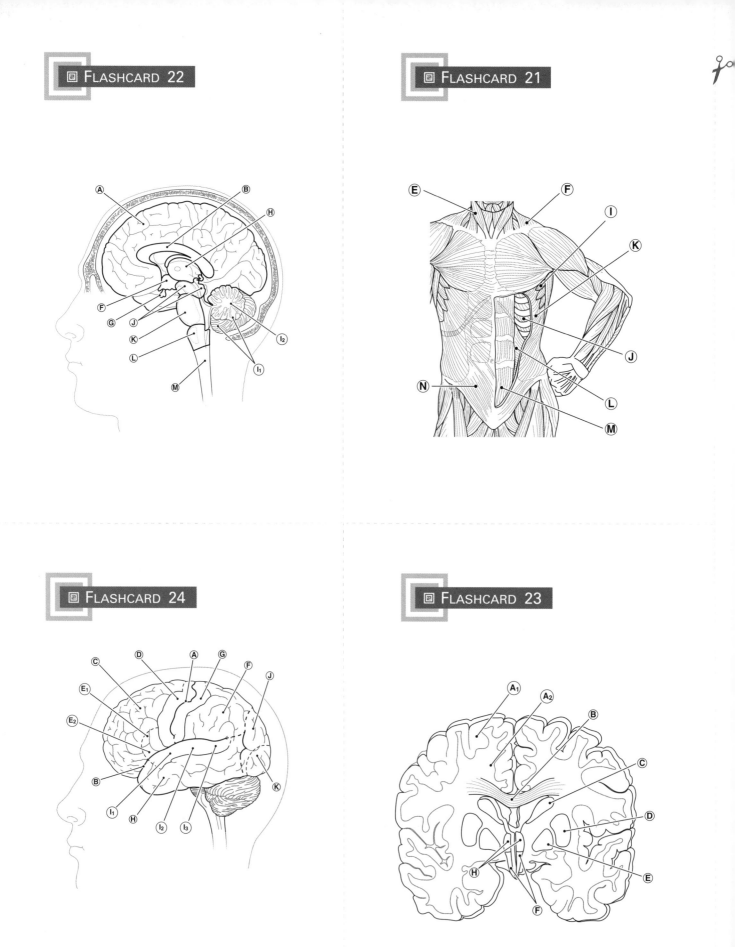

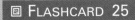
Coloring Exercise 5-9

- Ⓐ choroid plexus ◯
- Ⓑ lateral ventricles ◯
- Ⓒ third ventricle ◯
- Ⓓ interventricular foramina ◯
- Ⓔ fourth ventricle ◯
- Ⓕ cerebral aqueduct ◯
- Ⓖ central canal ◯
- Ⓗ subarachnoid space ◯
- Ⓘ arachnoid villi ◯
- Ⓙ superior sagittal sinus ◯
- Ⓚ straight sinus ◯

Coloring Exercise 5-10

- Ⓐ olfactory ◯
- Ⓑ optic ◯
- Ⓒ oculomotor ◯
- Ⓓ trochlear ◯
- Ⓔ trigeminal ◯
- Ⓕ abducens ◯
- Ⓖ facial ◯
- Ⓗ vestibulocochlear ◯
- Ⓘ glossopharyngeal ◯
- Ⓙ vagus ◯
- Ⓚ accessory ◯
- Ⓛ hypoglossal ◯

Coloring Exercise 6-2

- Ⓕ sclera ◯
- Ⓖ cornea ◯
- Ⓗ choroid ◯
- Ⓘ iris ◯
- Ⓘ₁ pupil ◯
- Ⓙ ciliary muscle ◯
- Ⓚ suspensory ligament ◯
- Ⓛ retina ◯
- Ⓛ₁ fovea centralis ◯
- Ⓜ optic nerve ◯
- Ⓟ lens ◯
- Ⓠ aqueous humor ◯
- Ⓡ vitreous body ◯
- Ⓢ conjunctiva ◯

Coloring Exercise 6-5

- Ⓑ external auditory canal ◯
- Ⓒ tympanic membrane ◯
- Ⓖ malleus ◯
- Ⓗ incus ◯
- Ⓘ stapes ◯
- Ⓙ vestibulocochlear nerve ◯
- Ⓚ semicircular canals ◯
- Ⓛ vestibule ◯
- Ⓜ cochlea ◯

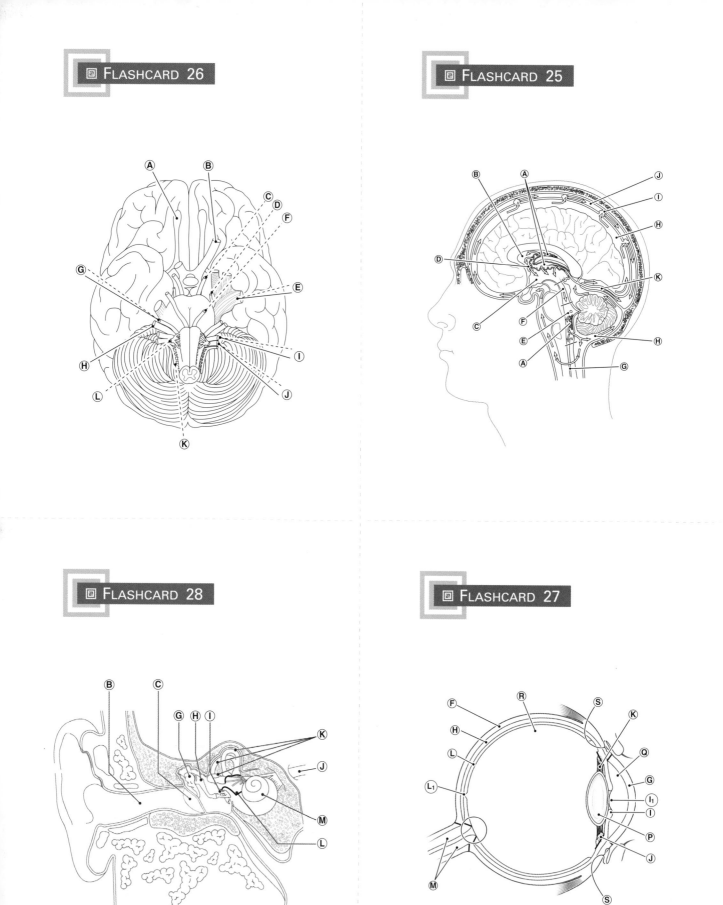

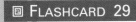

▣ Flashcard 29

Coloring Exercise 8-6

- Ⓐ superior vena cava ○
- Ⓑ inferior vena cava ○
- Ⓒ right atrium ○
- Ⓓ right AV valve ○
- Ⓔ right ventricle ○
- Ⓗ right pulmonary arteries ○
- Ⓛ right pulmonary vein ○
- Ⓤ endocardium ○
- Ⓥ myocardium ○
- Ⓦ epicardium ○

▣ Flashcard 30

Coloring Exercise 8-6

- Ⓕ pulmonary valve ○
- Ⓖ pulmonary trunk ○
- Ⓘ left pulmonary arteries ○
- Ⓜ left pulmonary vein ○
- Ⓝ left atrium ○
- Ⓞ left AV valve ○
- Ⓟ left ventricle ○
- Ⓠ aortic valve ○
- Ⓡ aorta ○
- Ⓢ chordae tendineae ○
- Ⓣ papillary muscle ○

▣ Flashcard 31

Coloring Exercise 8-9 (Arteries)

- Ⓐ ascending aorta ○
- Ⓑ aortic arch ○
- Ⓒ thoracic aorta ○
- Ⓕ coronary ○
- Ⓖ brachiocephalic ○
- Ⓗ right subclavian ○
- Ⓘ right common carotid ○
- Ⓙ left common carotid ○
- Ⓚ left subclavian ○
- Ⓛ intercostal ○

▣ Flashcard 32

Coloring Exercise 8-9 (Arteries)

- Ⓓ abdominal aorta ○
- Ⓔ common iliac ○
- Ⓜ celiac trunk ○
- Ⓝ hepatic ○
- Ⓞ splenic ○
- Ⓟ left gastric ○
- Ⓠ renal ○
- Ⓡ superior mesenteric ○
- Ⓢ gonadal ○
- Ⓣ inferior mesenteric ○
- Ⓤ external iliac ○
- Ⓥ internal iliac ○

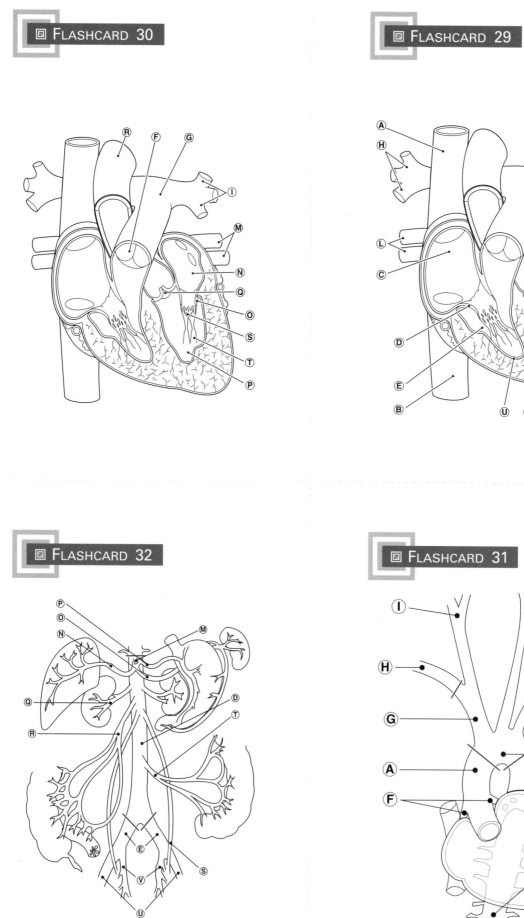

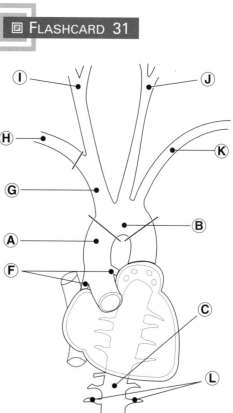

FLASHCARD 33

Coloring Exercise 8-10 (Arteries)

Ⓐ aortic arch ○
Ⓑ left common carotid ○
Ⓒ brachiocephalic ○
Ⓓ right common carotid ○
Ⓔ right subclavian ○
Ⓕ vertebral ○
Ⓖ axillary ○
Ⓗ brachial ○
Ⓘ radial ○
Ⓙ ulnar ○
Ⓚ volar arches ○
Ⓛ volar metacarpals ○
Ⓜ digitals ○

FLASHCARD 34

Coloring Exercise 8-10 (Arteries)

Ⓝ left common iliac ○
Ⓞ internal iliac ○
Ⓟ external iliac ○
Ⓠ femoral ○
Ⓡ deep femoral ○
Ⓢ popliteal ○
Ⓣ genicular ○
Ⓤ anterior tibial ○
Ⓥ dorsalis pedis ○
Ⓦ dorsal metatarsals ○
Ⓧ posterior tibial ○
Ⓨ peroneal ○

FLASHCARD 35

Coloring Exercise 8-11 (Arteries)

Ⓐ brachiocephalic trunk ○
Ⓑ right common carotid ○
Ⓒ right external carotid ○
Ⓓ superior thyroid ○
Ⓔ facial ○
Ⓕ labial ○
Ⓖ maxillary ○
Ⓗ superficial temporal ○
Ⓘ temporal ○
Ⓙ frontal ○
Ⓚ occipital ○
Ⓛ right subclavian ○
Ⓜ right vertebral ○
Ⓝ right internal carotid ○

FLASHCARD 36

Coloring Exercise 8-11 (Arteries)

Ⓜ right vertebral ○
Ⓝ right internal carotid ○
Ⓞ basilar ○
Ⓟ right posterior cerebral ○
Ⓠ right posterior communicating ○
Ⓡ right middle cerebral ○
Ⓢ right anterior cerebral ○
Ⓣ anterior communicating ○
Ⓤ left vertebral ○

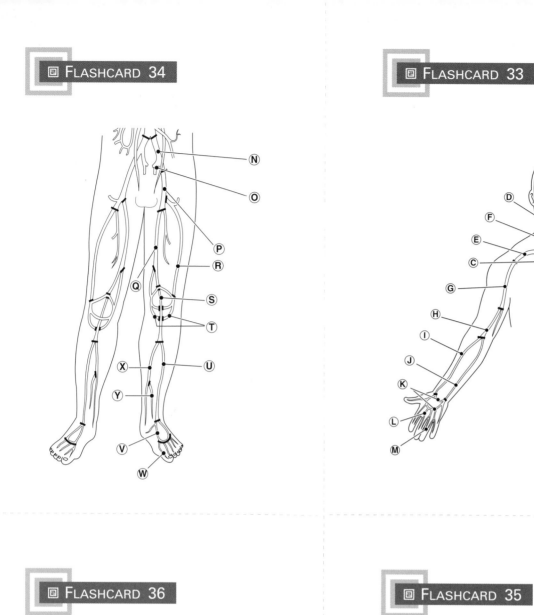

Ⓝ
Ⓞ
Ⓟ
Ⓡ
Ⓠ
Ⓢ
Ⓣ
Ⓤ
Ⓧ
Ⓨ
Ⓥ
Ⓦ

Ⓓ
Ⓕ
Ⓔ
Ⓒ
Ⓑ
Ⓐ
Ⓖ
Ⓗ
Ⓘ
Ⓙ
Ⓚ
Ⓛ
Ⓜ

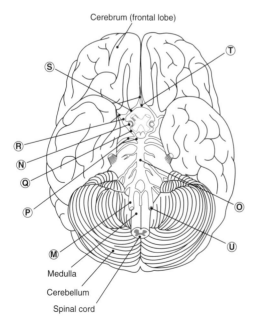

Cerebrum (frontal lobe)

Ⓣ
Ⓢ
Ⓡ
Ⓝ
Ⓠ
Ⓟ
Ⓞ
Ⓤ
Ⓜ

Medulla

Cerebellum

Spinal cord

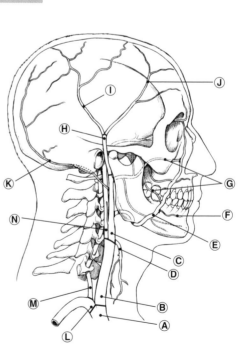

Ⓙ
Ⓘ
Ⓗ
Ⓚ
Ⓖ
Ⓕ
Ⓔ
Ⓒ
Ⓓ
Ⓝ
Ⓜ
Ⓑ
Ⓐ
Ⓛ

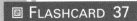
Coloring Exercise 8-12
(Veins)

- Ⓐ internal jugular ◯
- Ⓑ external jugular ◯
- Ⓒ brachiocephalic ◯
- Ⓓ superior vena cava ◯
- Ⓔ intercostal ◯
- Ⓕ azygos ◯
- Ⓖ volar digitalis ◯
- Ⓗ cephalic ◯
- Ⓘ basilic ◯
- Ⓙ median cubital ◯
- Ⓚ brachial ◯
- Ⓛ axillary ◯
- Ⓜ subclavian ◯

Coloring Exercise 8-13
(Veins)

- Ⓐ inferior vena cava ◯
- Ⓑ hepatic ◯
- Ⓒ renal ◯
- Ⓓ gonadal ◯
- Ⓔ lumbar ◯
- Ⓜ external iliac ◯
- Ⓝ internal iliac ◯
- Ⓞ right common iliac ◯
- Ⓟ left common iliac ◯

Coloring Exercise 8-13
(Veins)

- Ⓕ dorsal digitalis ◯
- Ⓖ venous arch ◯
- Ⓗ small saphenous ◯
- Ⓘ tibial ◯
- Ⓙ popliteal ◯
- Ⓚ femoral ◯
- Ⓛ great saphenous ◯

Coloring Exercise 8-14
(Veins)

- Ⓐ superficial temporal ◯
- Ⓑ external jugular ◯
- Ⓔ occipital ◯
- Ⓕ vertebral ◯
- Ⓖ inferior sagittal sinus ◯
- Ⓗ straight sinus ◯
- Ⓘ superior sagittal sinus ◯
- Ⓙ confluence ◯
- Ⓚ ophthalmic ◯
- Ⓛ cavernous sinus ◯
- Ⓜ petrosal sinuses ◯
- Ⓝ transverse sinus ◯
- Ⓞ facial ◯
- Ⓟ internal jugular ◯

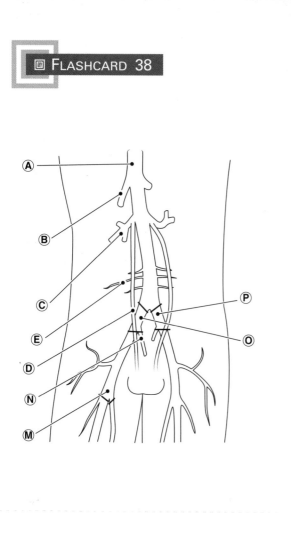

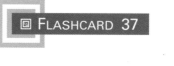
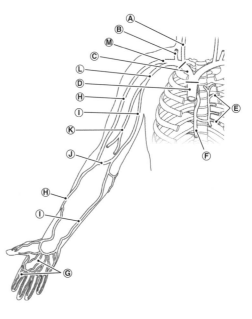

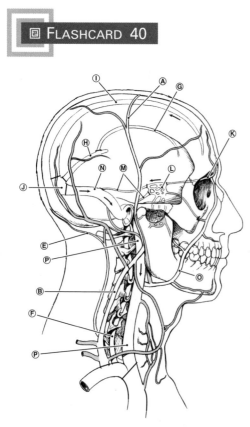

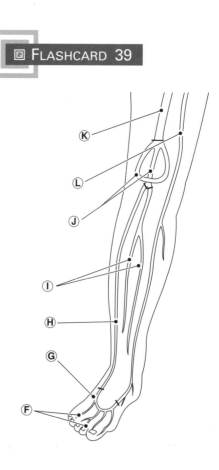